# STROKE
# SUPPORT
# & SURVIVAL
# GUIDE

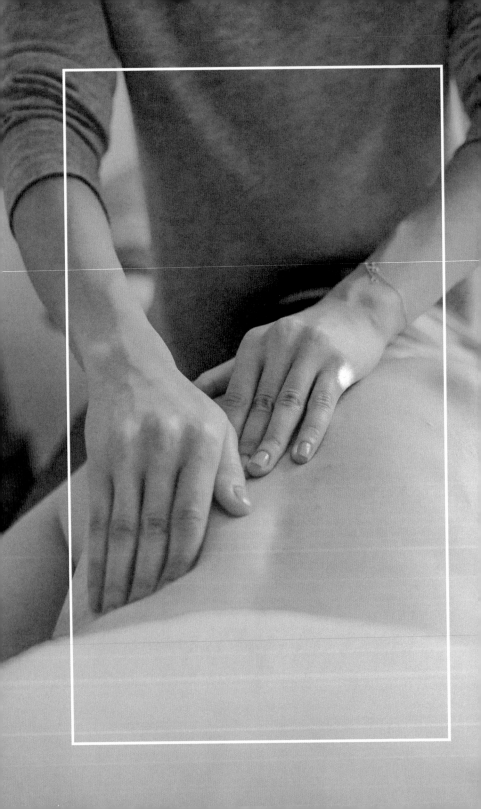

# STROKE SUPPORT & SURVIVAL GUIDE

THE SELF-HELP PLAN AND PERSONAL JOURNEY OF A HOLISTIC
PHYSICAL THERAPIST ASSISTANT AND HER FATHER

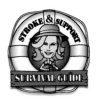

KATHI NAUMANN

## DEDICATION

This book is dedicated to the memory of my father, John Daniel Edwards, and to every adult son or daughter of a stroke survivor. If not for his life journey, this content would not exist. Dad, may your spirit live on in the pages of this book.

To the most amazing people I know: my husband Chris, and our children, Kylee and Mitchell, you three are unique individuals who have no boundaries, will truly accomplish great things, push my patience to the limits, and challenge me in ways I would never challenge myself. Thank you, Chris, Kylee, and Mitch for living this life with me.

To contact the publisher, visit www.strokeandsupport.com

To contact the author visit www.kathinaumann.com

ISBN - 978-0-578-59754-6

Printed in the United States of America

# TABLE OF CONTENTS

*For beautiful eyes, look for the good in others; for beautiful lips, speak only words of kindness; and for poise, walk with the knowledge you are never alone.*

Audrey Hepburn

# PREFACE

Being a caregiver has its challenges. Health care these days is confusing and over-whelming, with all the talk about Medicare changes, deductibles, explanation of benefits, social security, insurance benefits, denials, etc. An overload of confusing information can be nerve-wracking.

**Stroke Support & Survival Guide** is meant to be a comprehensive resource for caregivers of stroke victims.

In this guide, you will learn how to communicate effectively with medical staff, the importance of keeping a medical journal, what to look for in a rehabilitation setting, how to make thickened liquids and how to effectively integrate alternative medicine with conventional medicine to really heal a stroke survivor, how to make effective home modifications and how to think like a therapist.

It's based on decades of working one-on-one with people just like you and your stroke survivor from a caregiver's perspective and from a physical therapist as-sistant's perspective. You will learn how to effectively manage a person's medical care, think like a therapist and adopt caregiver self-care techniques. I've captured everything I have shown my rehabilitation clients and their family members and my personal experiences as a caregiver for a stroke victim parent in this book and designed it just for you, and me, the caregivers.

If you're a new caregiver who's ready to get serious and make positive changes in your life and the life of your loved one, then this guide is right for you.

This book reveals a step-by-step system to promote health and recovery for you and your survivor after stroke with a *touch of modern medicine meets holistic medicine* approach. You'll learn how to turn your fear into confidence and gain the knowledge that supports you, the caregiver, concerned family member, or friend to promote a more ideal lifestyle and improve the health of your stroke survivor.

This survival guide is designed to be taken with you wherever you go. Write and document everything. It will save you time and even money down the road. It will help you to remember important dates as well as medication changes and reactions. Looking for a rehab? Don't fret—this survival guide will navigate you through the process and open your eyes to the world of recovery.

**Stroke Support & Survival Guide** includes:

- What to do first when someone you love has a stroke
- Ways to keep yourself organized and turn your fear into confidence for concise, clear communication with medical staff
- Easy-to-follow instructions
- Recipes for brain-health smoothies
- Home modification solutions
- Medical journal organization tips
- What to look for in a rehab, along with printable graphics so you "get it" immediately
- How to avoid wasted time and energy on figuring out all this stuff and spend that life-saving time with your loved one
- Access to free exercise and transfer videos
- How to build strength and promote vitality in your stroke survivor and begin the self-help process

I wrote this guide to help you avoid all the heartache, headaches, & hiccups caregivers experience. I hope you find it helpful in navigating the challenging times ahead.

# INTRODUCTION

Our children were four and five years old. It was a Sunday night when I finally sat down for a quiet moment when I realized something: "Chris, I don't feel well. Something isn't quite right. I am nervous, uneasy - something is wrong." I had a feeling that something bad was happening somewhere but I just couldnt figure it out.

On that very sad September day in 2001, I woke up early, washed some laundry, and was hanging it on the clothesline. I recognized the stillness and quietness around me, and decided to sit down to take it all in under the large gum tree that provided a pillar for one end of my clothesline. I had no idea that something beyond my belief was happening to our country. I just knew I had an uneasy feeling, and I felt it again on September 5, 2005.

The phone rang around two in the morning, and as my husband and I scrambled to find the phone, we missed the call. Then we heard a helicopter fly over our house. I sat straight up in bed and said, "Something is really wrong." My mother was trying to call us to tell us that Dad was being flown to Shock Trauma in Baltimore, Maryland, but I didn't know that because when I called back no one answered the phone. I threw some clothes on and drove straight to my parents' house just in time to see the helicopter take off.

We drove almost two hours to the hospital to find our father lying on a gurney with a young doctor looking over him, asking him to remove his plate. At that point in time, Dad was able to help take out his plate using his left hand. I remember turning to the young doctor and saying, "Please be aggressive." He turned to me and replied, "We always are."

There we were, my brother, sister, mother, and I, standing in the hallway of a dimly lit emergency room. We could hear sirens in the distance. It was as though we were in another world. We stood there dumbfounded as we watched the curtain being pulled around Dad and the emergency medical team, then sadly found our way to the waiting room.

Our mother asked us all to pray, and I remember thinking to myself, "What the heck is that going to do for us?" As she prayed for Dad to survive, I prayed for him to pass away. Maybe that sounds harsh, but at that point I knew that he was probably having a stroke, and if he were to survive, he would live a life of pure hell. I obviously had a lot to learn about the power of prayer. Dad survived a massive stroke, one we later learned most people don't survive. I guess he was lucky? It was later in this journey that I realized that I was actually the lucky one.

Unfortunately, the young doctor had not made the best decision, and our father was not given the TPn blood clot-busting medication that would have stopped or at least slowed down the stroke, and he continued to stroke over the next three days. He stayed in ICU for those three days and then was transferred to a "regular" hospital room. That's when it all started…

Dad was trying to read the ticker on the bottom of the television screen and was confused as to why the news was chopping off half the sentence. I'll never forget that moment. It was then I realized his eyes had been affected by the stroke. The nurse walked in around that time, and I can still see in my mind's eye the look of concern on her face.

Dad suffered from homonymous hemianopsia. It is estimated that 70 percent of the injuries leading to homonymous hemianopsia are due to a blockage in the brain, and males from the age fifty to seventy are the most affected. Dad was sixty. When he looked at a clock, he saw the numbers 1 through 6 only, and the other side of the clock was black. He could only see half of his world. Because of that, he sat in his chair with his upper body turned ninety degrees to the right. Can you imagine how we felt when we realized that he couldn't find a piece of paper in front of him, no less try to read it? We were devastated. At that moment I realized that driving was no longer an option, reading would be a major challenge, and teaching him to sit facing forward in a chair was now our starting point.

Eight years of recovery brought tears, smiles, and a wonderful opportunity for me to really get to know my father. When I was a teenager, my father was a closet alcoholic. I would find half-gallon bottles of Canadian Mist in the most unusual places: the wood stove, between bushel baskets in the garage. We had a horrible relationship, as you can imagine. My high school graduation was probably the straw that broke the camel's back for me. He showed up so drunk that he could barely stand up. I hated him. I really never had any desire to give him a chance to redeem himself after he got sober. I felt he had robbed me of my innocence. The emotions I felt back then were paralyzing. I was forced to grow up fast and make adult decisions. I felt alone.

Those feelings have also crept into my adult life, sometimes with a vengeance. Now, you could look at my life and wonder why I would ever feel alone. I have a large biological family with deep roots in my hometown going back 400 years. My husband also has a huge family, and we have many truly amazing friends that we call our family. I am truly grateful for my life, yet sometimes I still feel alone and that I have to "do this life" on my own. It's weird to me how we are all shaped by the experiences we had as children.

Enough about me. Let's get back to why I wrote this book in the first place. As time went on, Dad and I became really good friends, believe it or not. I learned about how sensitive and caring he was and how much he actually loved his family. He especially loved children and helping others that may be having a hard time traveling down the road of life. He was truly a special person, and I am grateful that I got to know him.

After all the rehab stays, hospitalizations, and running to doctors, life started to settle down. Some days all we could do was talk, and he would ask me, "Why do you think this happened to me?" My thought at first was that he/we were being punished, but as time went on I realized that my father's stroke was a lesson to us all. Most of all I learned that had my father's stroke never happened, I would have never gotten to know the gentle, kindhearted man that always thought of others before himself. All the sacrifices I made, the time away from my own family to spend time with him, didn't make me rich, didn't make me a star, but what it did do was bring me emotions. Those emotions made me stronger when his time got shorter, and now I can look back on those hard times and smile, because I have peace and am proud that I did the most I could do to help someone in need: my dad.

I am writing this book because I feel like I need to share my experience with the world. We endured so much, and I hope that I can shelter someone else's family from the heartache, if only a little bit. I feel I owe it to my father and to my husband and children to complete this project. I took time away from them to create the content for this survival guide and I appreciate all the sacrifices they made during that time.

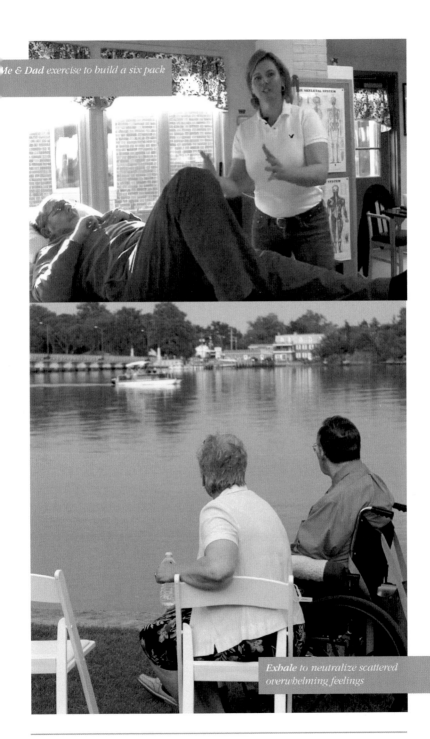

Me & Dad exercise to build a six pack

Exhale to neutralize scattered overwhelming feelings

# THE STROKE RECOVERY JOURNEY: AN OVERVIEW

When a loved one has a stroke, there are typically five stages of the recovery process, which we'll cover in depth in this guide:

1. The Emergency Room (ER)
2. The Hospital
3. Short-Term (Acute Care) Rehabilitation
4. Long-Term (Skilled Nursing) Rehabilitation
5. Home Healthcare

The Emergency Room will stabilize your loved one. They will start the testing to make a definite diagnosis.

The Hospital is the next venue to recover enough to make the plans for the next level of care. The hospital rehab team typically consists of a discharge planner, speech therapist, physical therapist, and occupational therapist.

Acute-Care Rehabilitation is where a patient receives active but short-term medical treatment. Rehabilitation for stroke survivors typically begins in a rehabilitation facility: this is where the stroke survivor relearns basic skills such as talking, eating, dressing, and walking. Some larger hospital systems have certified stroke centers. State that you'd like your loved one to go to an acute rehabilitation hospital or a stroke center. This will often allow your stroke survivor a little more time in rehabilitation. An average acute rehab stay is twenty days.

Long-Term Rehabilitation is the next step. Long-term care rehabilitation is sustained care in a long-term care/skilled nursing facility that may be in a nursing home. If you have not yet called your insurance company, this is the time to do it. Find out exactly what your policy states about rehabilitation. Skilled/long-term rehabilitation can include nursing, physical therapy, occupational therapy, speech therapy, and respiratory therapy. This is where your loved one will increase their strength, flexibility, and endurance. Ultimately, this is the place where the patient can begin to regain their independence. I have learned that most people want to go home and don't always have a good grasp on the reality of what just happened to them and their deficits. Sometimes you have to exhibit some "tough love" and encourage your loved one to go to a rehab center.

Home Care is an option if the stroke is very small, sometimes called a transient ischemic attack (TIA). TIAs typically leave the stroke survivor with very few symptoms, which is great. However, it must also be seen as a wake-up call that something is very wrong and that there may be more to come. Going home after a TIA does not mean your loved one can go off on their own. It means that they need medical attention, and there may be mild cognitive deficits that are a little harder to see at first glance. If your loved one is headed home, then you will need to make some modifications to make sure it's safe and supports the recovery process. See chapter 5 for everything you need to know about home modifications.

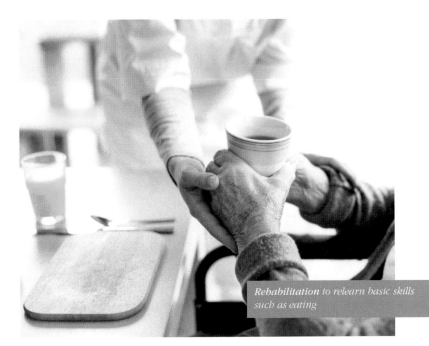

*Rehabilitation to relearn basic skills such as eating*

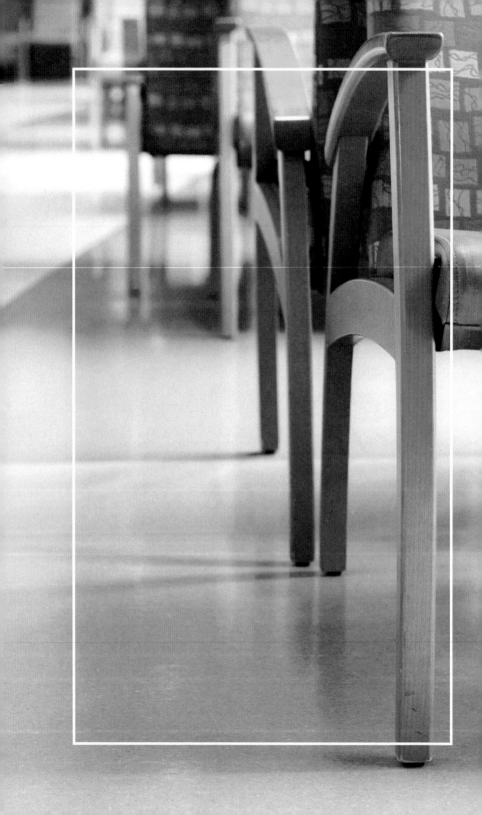

# CHAPTER 1

# THE EMERGENCY ROOM

*I wrote this chapter as a result of my own experience of sitting in the ER waiting to hear the news about my father, when I could have used someone telling me to get grounded and to breathe. There's a chance you're reading this after having already spent hours in the emergency room in the wake of your loved one's stroke, in which case some of the events I describe may have already occurred to you. Even still, I hope that the advice in this chapter is still helpful as you continue on the rollercoaster of post-stroke care and recovery. And if you happen to be reading this chapter as a way of being prepared for the hopefully unlikely possibility of someone you love having a stroke, then I hope of course that you will never have to use my advice. But in the slim chance that you do ever need it, I hope it is of some use and comfort to you.*

## WHAT'S HAPPENING?

A stroke is a "brain attack." It occurs when a clot blocks the blood supply to the brain or when a blood vessel in the brain bursts, also called an aneurysm or hemorrhagic stroke. Either way, the brain is deprived of needed oxygen. Treatment usually begins in the ER, and the caregiver's role begins right away.

## CLEAR YOUR HEAD AND GET GROUNDED

You are about to experience a rollercoaster ride of emotions. For some, the rollercoaster is only small little bunny hills, and for some (like us) the rollercoaster ride swoops deep down under the water's surface.

There really isn't much time to wrap your head around what's happening, and that's why it's super-important to find a place to take a break. Go outside if possible. Spend a few minutes away from the chaos. Tell someone exactly where you will be in case the medical team is looking for you, and then go outside the hospital to take a break from the overwhelming smells, lights, and hustle of the hospital setting. Take a moment to take a few deep breaths and calm yourself down. Find a bench, sit up, and place both your feet on the ground. Put your feet directly on the earth if possible. Grounding or earthing is a technique that uses the Earth's energy to heal the human body and soul. Grounding and healing the body for just a few minutes may make a huge difference in how you respond to any situation. A significant life-changing event can throw us off balance, and grounding has been proven to bring us back into balance. If you are feeling overwhelmed, try it.

Next, sit up, take a deep breath, and fill your belly with air. Calm your mind for a moment. Focus your attention on the color you see when you close your eyes. Clearing your mind for even one minute may be the only thing you're able to give back to yourself all day. Living in a state of constant arousal keeps the body in long-term stress: we become overly alert to force our emotions toward focusing on changing the outcome of the situation. The more you focus on the stroke survivor, the hospital, and the moment, the less energy you have for internal thoughts and emotions, causing your body to become out of balance, and then you can become resentful. It's going to take energy to break the resentment, fear, and external focus and shift your attention from the outside world to your inside world. It's very important to take a few minutes for yourself to overcome survival mode and create enough energy to create and design a new destiny. Get ready, because certain areas of your life may fall apart. That's okay. Let them. Don't try to put your old life back together yet: try to understand that this tragedy is creating space for something new.

Breathe. The very first thing we do is take a breath, and the very last thing we do is take a breath. I'd say that breathing must be pretty important. Take the time to breathe now. Breathe in through your nose and exhale out of your mouth. When you blow out the air, push the air out starting with your diaphragm and squeeze your heart then close your throat. This type of deep breathing helps to reset and recharge your energy.

Now that you've cleared your head a bit, there are a few things you need to think about:

1. **Advocate.** It's your job to let the doctors know that you think your loved one has had a stroke. It's important to tell the back story: have you noticed any changes lately, such as sleeping more, dizziness, or headaches? If you're the timid, shy type, now is not the time to step into the background. Everyone needs support (even the doctor), and that includes you, the caregiver, but now is the time to support your loved one. Give the doctor as much information about your loved one's symptoms as possible. Have a family member or friend bring you their medications and make a list.[1] Stroke victims are unable to make sound decisions when undergoing such a traumatic experience, and sometimes the stroke is severe, leaving them unable to communicate at all.

2. **Tell the whole story.** As the saying goes, hindsight is 20/20, and this is not the time to feel guilty. Did your loved one show signs you didn't act on? Please don't feel bad; it's not your fault. Maybe you did push your loved one to go to the doctor, and maybe you didn't. It's okay. It's water under the bridge now. That was in the past, and now it's time to move forward.

3. **Be assertive.** Make sure the patient is seen within five minutes of arriving at the ER. There's a saying with strokes: "Time lost is brain lost." If you need to make a scene, so be it, but there's a right and wrong way to communicate. Stay calm, but be assertive by asking when your loved one will be seen. There are times when a blood clot-busting medication called tissue plasminogen activator (tPA) might be warranted, but there is a time frame (three hours) in which this can be administered. Being assertive might give your loved one time, which makes way for options and less brain damage.

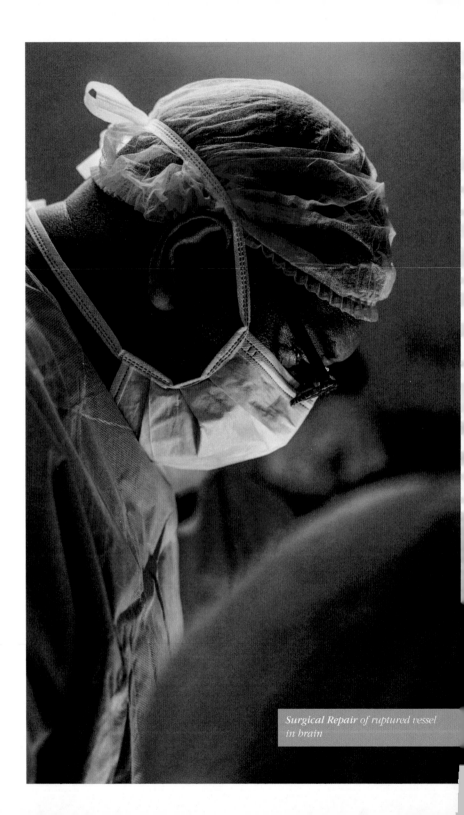

*Surgical Repair* of ruptured vessel in brain

**4. Understand the brain tests.** The doctor will order a brain scan that will show which part of the brain has been damaged and whether it was caused by a clot or bleed. This should be done within an hour of arriving at the hospital for those who are experiencing an acute (sudden-onset) stroke. Let's hope that it's done right away so that a sound and definitive diagnosis can be made. There are tests that the ER team will perform right away. Go to the end of this chapter to get a full understanding of what these tests are.

- Physical examination
- Blood tests
- Computerized tomography (CT or CAT scan)
- Magnetic resonance imaging (MRI)
- Carotid ultrasound
- Cerebral angiogram
- Echo cardiogram

**5. Ask questions.** Find out the type of stroke and the treatment that will be given. This is where you will need to consider getting a notebook to have everything at your fingertips. There are some great resources at Kathinaumann.com to help with this, but for now just get a notebook and start writing. Write down your questions and thoughts, as well as other's thoughts and conversations with the medical staff. To help you in knowing what to ask, here's some information about the different types of strokes and how they're treated.

There are three types of stroke:
- Ischemic (clotting)
- Hemorrhagic (bleeding, also known as an aneurysm or brain bleed)
- Transient ischemic attack (TIA, also known as a mini-stroke)

Strokes are similar to heart attacks, and the two are sometimes confused. Strokes are given less attention than heart attacks, but both involve a cut-off of blood supply. In a heart attack, the blood supply to the heart and then all other organs is cut off. In a stroke, the blood supply is cut off to the brain from an ischemic (blood clot) stroke or a hemorrhagic (bleeding) stroke.

An ischemic stroke is caused by a blood clot blocking a blood vessel.

A hemorrhagic stroke (brain bleed) is caused by bleeding of blood vessels of the brain either directly into the brain parenchyma or into the subarachnoid space surrounding brain tissue.

In terms of treatment, generally, a person who is treated within three hours of experiencing a stroke—specifically an ischemic stroke (one caused by a blood clot in the brain)—has a 30 percent greater chance of recovering with no or little debilitating effects.[2]

- TPn
- Endovascular procedures
- Surgical treatment

**6. Call in support.** Identify people who will serve as the family's spokesperson, investigator, and researcher.

**Spokesperson:** This individual will be responsible for sharing information with family members and close friends. This is very important. That way you text one person the updates and that person sends out the information to family and friends. Energy conservation is key. Conserving your energy and keeping yourself healthy is vital to the recovery process. If you need a break, take it.

**Investigator:** One very important job to give someone is to start investigating rehabilitation centers. This might seem premature, but trust me, it's not. Healthcare is a business set out to make a profit. The faster the pace of the process, the more money will be made for the hospital. You'd think that it works the opposite, right? You would think that the longer your loved one stays in the hospital the more money the hospital makes. It doesn't work that way. The reimbursement rate goes down each day the patient is in the hospital. The whole process is fast-paced and overwhelming so let's get prepared.

If you live in a large city, it's much easier to decide on a rehab, as there are stroke centers and multiple rehab centers to choose from. If you live in the country, like us, choosing a rehab can be overwhelming. The main focus, though, is on the patient. What is the best location for the patient, not the caregivers. The Rehab section of this book will tell you exactly what to look for in a rehab and how the whole process works.

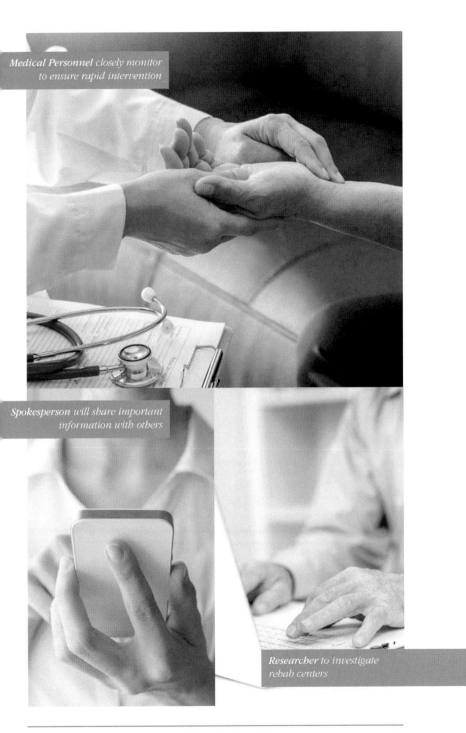

*Medical Personnel* closely monitor to ensure rapid intervention

*Spokesperson* will share important information with others

*Researcher* to investigate rehab centers

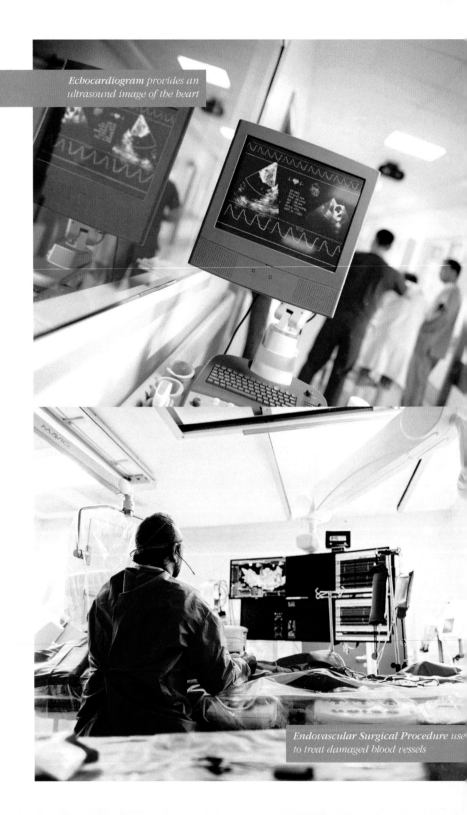

*Echocardiogram provides an ultrasound image of the heart*

*Endovascular Surgical Procedure used to treat damaged blood vessels*

**Researcher:** Have someone sign your name and email up for stroke-related newsletters from the following sources. These newsletters are full of information that will give you hope. Stay positive and think positive.

- www.stroke.org
- www.cdc.gov/stroke
- www.strokefoundation.org
- www.strokeconnection.org
- www.eso-stroke.org

## TESTS AND PROCEDURES

Your stroke patient may be given a number of tests and procedures. Here are the main ones.

- **Physical examination.** The doctor will ask you, the caregiver, what symptoms the stroke survivor has been having, when they started, and what they were doing when the symptoms began. The doctor then will evaluate whether these symptoms are still present. They will want to know what medications your loved one takes and if they have experienced any head injuries. You'll be asked about the personal and family history of heart disease, transient ischemic attack (TIA), and stroke. The blood pressure will be measured, and they will listen to the heart for a whooshing sound (bruit) over the neck (carotid) arteries, which may indicate atherosclerosis. The doctor may also use an ophthalmoscope to check for signs of tiny cholesterol crystals or clots in the blood vessels at the back of the patient's eyes.
- **Blood tests.** They may have several blood tests, which tell the care team how fast their blood clots, whether the blood sugar is abnormally high or low, whether critical blood chemicals are out of balance, or whether the patient may have an infection. Managing the blood's clotting time and levels of sugar and other key chemicals will be part of stroke care.
- **Carotid ultrasound.** Sound waves create detailed images of the inside of the carotid arteries in the neck. This test shows buildup of fatty deposits (plaques) and blood flow in your carotid arteries.
- **Cerebral angiogram.** The doctor inserts a thin, flexible tube (catheter) through a small incision, usually in the groin, and guides it through the major arteries and into the carotid or vertebral artery. Then the doctor injects a dye into the blood vessels

to make them visible under X-ray imaging. This procedure gives a detailed view of the arteries in the patient's brain and neck.

- **Computerized tomography (CT or CAT) scan.** A CT scan uses a series of X-rays to create a detailed image of the brain. A CT scan can show a hemorrhage, tumor, stroke and other conditions. Doctors may inject a dye into the bloodstream to view the blood vessels in the neck and brain in greater detail (computerized tomography angiography). Your doctor may use different types of CT scans depending on your situation.

- **Echocardiogram.** Uses sound waves to create detailed images of the heart. An echocardiogram can find a source of clots in the heart that may have traveled from the heart to the brain and caused the stroke.

- **Endovascular procedures.** Endovascular procedures may be used to treat certain hemorrhagic strokes. The doctor inserts a long tube through a major artery in the leg or arm and then guides the tube to the site of the weak spot or break in a blood vessel. The tube is then used to install a device, such as a coil, to repair the damage or prevent bleeding.

- **Surgical treatment.** Hemorrhagic strokes may be treated with surgery. If the bleeding is caused by a ruptured aneurysm, a metal clip may be put in place to stop the blood loss.

- **Magnetic resonance imaging (MRI).** Uses powerful radio waves and magnets to create a detailed view of the brain. An MRI can detect brain tissue damaged by an ischemic stroke and brain hemorrhages. The doctor may inject a dye into a blood vessel to view the arteries and veins and highlight blood flow (magnetic resonance angiography, or magnetic resonance venography).

- **Transesophageal echocardiogram.** A flexible tube with a small device (transducer) is sent through the throat and down into the tube that connects the back of the mouth to the stomach (esophagus). The esophagus is directly behind the heart. A transesophageal echocardiogram can create clear, detailed ultrasound images of the heart and any blood clots.

---

[1] You can download and print a form from www.kathinaumann.com.

[2] www.cdc.gov/stroke/treatments.htm

---

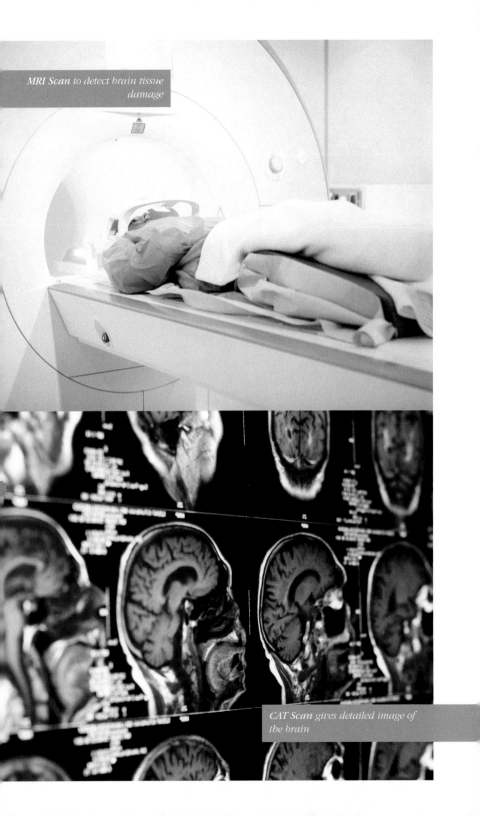

MRI Scan to detect brain tissue damage

CAT Scan gives detailed image of the brain

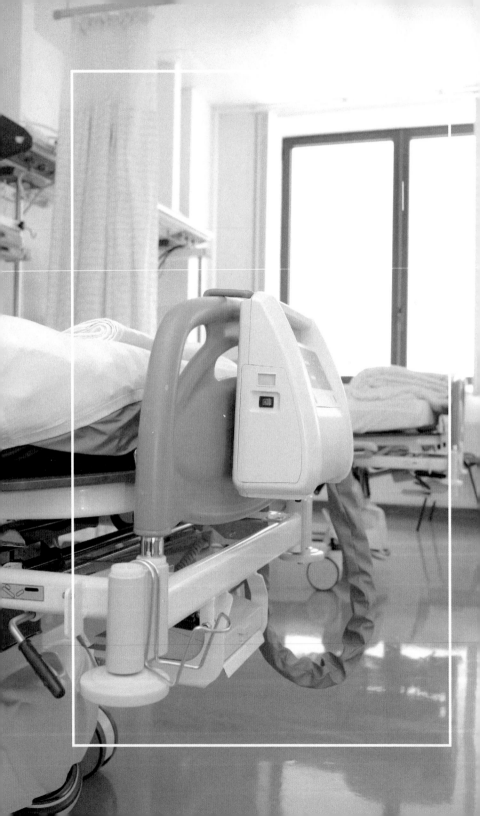

# CHAPTER 2

# THE HOSPITAL

*Once your stroke survivor has been stabilized in the Emergency Room, they will be given a hospital bed. The hospital room becomes home for about three to six days (sometime longer for patients with hemorrhagic strokes). The hospital stay is a fast-paced experience where many important decisions will have to be made. The discharge planner, sometimes called the care coordinator, will be knocking on your door soon. You may be feeling a bit overwhelmed, wondering why discharge planning is being discussed already, but it is a necessary discussion that needs to be addressed. Be patient, be an open listener, and write things down.*

They will be carrying forms for you to fill out called **advanced directives**. Our father was sixty years old when he had his stroke, and these forms were probably something he thought he'd get around to doing one day. If your loved one does not have a living will, traditionally the health care providers will turn to you for the answers. Are you ready to make a decision about someone else's life? If the patient does not have a do-not-resuscitate (DNR) order in place, the caregiver may have to decide on life-saving measures.This is the first of many difficult decisions you will have to make. Make the decision and do not regret the decision that you made. Do not second-guess yourself. Do your best, and that will be good enough.

## LOOKING AFTER THE PATIENT

Medical personnel should closely monitor the patient to ensure rapid intervention if another stroke or complication occurs. Once the type of stroke has been diagnosed, the patient will be given more tests to determine what caused the stroke and what effects the stroke has had. Some of these tests will include:

- **Swallowing test.** Difficulty swallowing is most common immediately after a stroke, but usually declines over time. Known as dysphagia, it's a paralysis of the throat muscle that can make eating, drinking, taking medicine, and breathing difficult. It can also lead to complications such as chest infections or pneumonia.
- **Mobility assessment.** Members of the stroke team will assess the patient physically and determine what help they will need to position themselves and move around.
- **Pressure area risk assessment.** Pressure ulcers or bed sores result from decreased ability to move and pressure on areas of the body because of immobility.
- **Continence assessment.** It's common for stroke survivors to experience continence issues, but there are ways to manage these issues.
- **Communication and cognitive assessments.** These tests will determine whether the stroke caused issues that have made it difficult for the patient to talk or understand and process information. There are a variety of ways to address these issues, as well.
- **Nutritional and hydration status.** These tests will ensure that the patient isn't becoming dehydrated and is taking in the proper nutrients.

A treatment regimen will be assigned to reduce stroke-related complications and help patients obtain the best possible functional outcome.

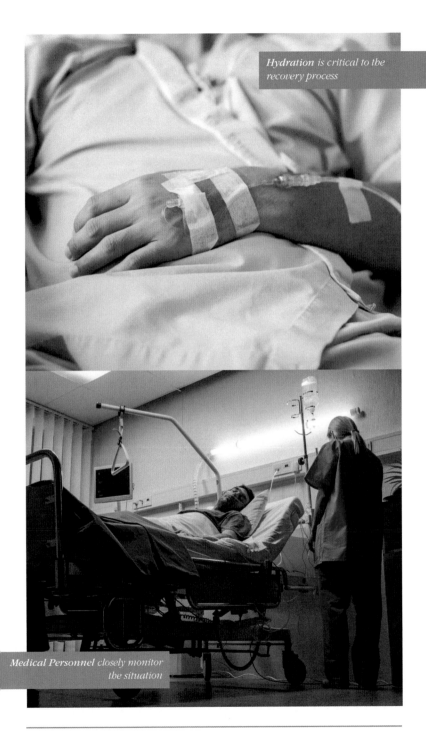

*Hydration* is critical to the recovery process

*Medical Personnel* closely monitor the situation

## THE CAREGIVER: LOOK AFTER YOU AND GET ORGANIZED

Make arrangements for yourself. What will your schedule be like? Where are you staying? Many times, large hospital systems have houses where family members can stay for extended periods of time. These houses are close to the hospital and typically offer hot meals, laundry facilities and a place to rest. To find out more, ask your Care Coordinator or the front desk person. I think most people are good and want to help. Accept the help while you are going through the hardest part of your life then pay it forward when you can. Love will get you through.

Now, it's time to get organized.

**1. Start a medical journal.** A lot of information will be coming at you quickly from tests galore, results, and diagnosis to treatments, medications, and names and titles of the stroke team. A medical journal is one of the most essential tools you'll use. It contains the personal health records of the patient in one place. It allows you to communicate effectively with medical personnel and get the best possible care for your stroke survivor. I can't stress enough how important it is to stay organized, and a medical journal will save precious time and energy. If creating a journal seems too much right now, it's very important to keep track of the medications taken prior to the stroke and then the medications that are prescribed at each level of the rehab process. This will cut down the risk of medical mistakes.

My father was having odd symptoms that were brought up at a random care plan meeting (which you can read more about later in this chapter). Ironically, the dietitian figured out that Dad was being overdosed on a heart medication. He survived this medical mistake, but it's very possible that if that dietician had not picked up on the medication mistake, he would have died. We learned a harsh but valuable lesson from the situation: Keeping clear medical records is imperative to the recovery process.

For more information on how to keep a medical journal or to download medical journal forms go to www.kathinaumann.com. You'll also find a sample medical journal in the appendix.

**2. Contact the insurance company.** Ask the representative to clarify what type of plan your loved one has, what services are covered, and the procedures that must be followed to receive all the coverage the patient deserves. When insurance companies deny payment for medical services, it's often because the consumer didn't follow the required procedures or failed to understand the limits of coverage. On the other hand, you may learn of unexpected benefits the plan offers, such as support groups and classes. Document the name of the case worker at the insurance company who has been assigned to your case. If they have not assigned someone, ask the insurance company if you can have a contact person. Keep lines of communication open with that person.

3. **Learn basic nursing skills.** There are basic skills that will be helpful if you are able and know how to perform them. Nurses can instruct you on:

- **Avoiding pressure sores.** When someone is consistently positioned on their back, there are certain pressure points on the body that are susceptible to sores. Heels, hips, low back, shoulder blades, hips, and ankles are at highest risk, especially the heels. Place a rolled blanket or heels-up cushion under the ankle/calf areas to keep the heels off the bed.
- **Performing wheelchair transfers.** Watch and ask questions when your loved one is being transferred from one surface to another. Healthcare workers are sometimes very focused on the patient and forget about teaching the family and friends about the safest way to transfer their loved one. Some venues frown upon family members transferring patients, so you may want to ask and respect the professional opinion of the therapists. The last thing anyone wants is to put your loved one in harm's way.
- **Dealing with bowel or bladder incontinence.** A stroke sometimes shocks the whole body system, leaving the survivor unable to control their bowel and bladder. Incontinence is typically embarrassing for the patient. The earlier the client is placed on a bowel and bladder schedule, the better. Sometimes the simple act of having a schedule can reprogram the brain and body to work together.
- **Dietary needs.** A nutritionist can help you plan for dietary needs. If your loved one has swallowing issues, it's important to work with a speech therapist to learn how to make thickened liquids.
- **Massage.** Rub or massage the affected side. Massaging the affected side of a stroke survivor helps to bring awareness and blood flow that have healing effects. Read more in chapter 6.

4. **Prepare for the next step:** Home or rehab. Ready! Set! Go! The process of getting your loved one out of the hospital and on to the next venue is very fast. In my

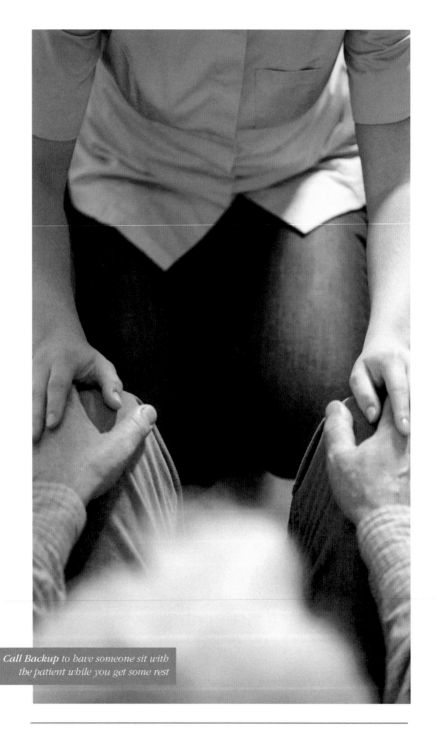

*Call Backup to have someone sit with the patient while you get some rest*

opinion, the entire American healthcare system is based on financial gain, placing the patient's needs at the back, but healthcare is slowly changing. I hope that your loved one is fortunate enough to live in an area that embraces functional medicine and complementary and alternative medicine. The integrative medical model and family model tend to be more compassionate and caring.

**5. Call in backup.** Self-care begins now. You can't assist your stroke survivor if you are sick. Delegate tasks to all the people who ask you if you need anything. Take breaks, and have someone sit with the patient while you get some rest. When you are completely clear and focused on the outcome you want, you will rewire your brain and prime it for what can happen in the future. Focusing on the future and creating strong mental energy requires some personal time, so plan ten minutes every day to imagine a positive day while you rehearse what you need to do that day.

## THE IMPORTANCE OF THINKING LIKE A THERAPIST

When your loved one is in the hospital, you need to step up to your role as their advocate and adopt a therapist's mindset if you want to ensure the best outcome for them. There are a couple of important nutrition and hygiene guidelines you'll need to follow right away. I also want to share some tips on how to interact and communicate with the doctors and clinical staff to ensure your loved one gets the best care and nothing gets lost between the cracks.

## THERAPY FOR YOUR LOVED ONE: #1 FOOD ADDITIVE TO AVOID AT ALL COST

The hospital is a great place to start thinking about your loved one's healing plan. A stroke affects the brain, obviously, and we need to support brain health.

With that in mind, let's talk about high fructose corn syrup (HFCS). HFCS is a by-product of corn. It was introduced into the food market back in the 70s when tariffs were placed on sugar imports and food manufacturers were looking for a cheap alternative to sugar. There is evidence that shows HFCS is the key to understanding the rising obesity rate in the US.

HFCS can also be contaminated with mercury. Mercury is a neurotoxin, which means that it is toxic to our nervous system. One of the side effects of mercury is anxiety, and guess what the number one mental health diagnosis is in the US? Anxiety.

HFCS can sometimes be found in feeding tube nutrition and saline solutions that are sweetened with glucose, calorie-enhanced Jell-O, and other products that boost nutrition. Nutrition for the brain is critical and keeping clear of HFCS is extremely important for you and your loved one's brain health.

What do you do if the medications have HFCS? If the container does not have the ingredient list, ask to see the label. Ask for an alternative.

## THERAPY FOR YOUR LOVED ONE: MOUTH HYGIENE

Digestion actually starts in the mouth. It is where the saliva starts to break down the food. Keeping the mouth clean is critical to our health and especially to someone whose health has been compromised. Most hospitals have swabs that can be used to help clean the mouth of someone who is unable to brush their teeth, but sometimes these swabs are flavored with artificial sweeteners and flavors. It's probably not a good idea to introduce more toxins in the body, and a great reason to make your own. Ask the nurse for some swabs. They look like a lollipop with foam on the end. Squeeze the juice of ½ a lemon or lime into a small jar and mix with equal amounts of water to create a lemon water solution. Tighten down with a lid so it doesn't spill during transport and you are all set.

Lemons have a multitude of benefits, from preserving food to cleaning to medicine. In particular:

- **Rich in vitamin C, which is needed for many reactions in our bodies. A lack of vitamin C can lead to fatigue, stress-related problems and a weakened immune system, so it is really important to include it in your loved ones' (and your) diet.**
- **Natural antihistamine and play a role in preventing allergies and inflammation, and also contain antiviral properties and act as an antibiotic.**
- **Pectin, which can help with reducing cholesterol.**
- **Calcium, which helps create stronger, healthier teeth and bones.**
- **Citric acid, an alkalizing substance that helps to decrease acidity in the body.[3]**

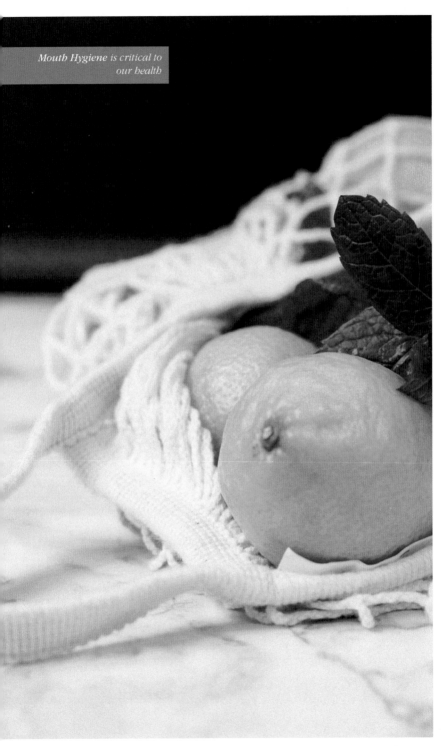

## THERAPY AND ADVOCACY FOR YOUR LOVED ONE: EFFECTIVE COMMUNICATION

Now that we have stated the importance of avoiding HFCS and practicing mouth care, let's talk about communication.

In this fast-paced world, don't be upset when the doctor runs in and out of your loved one's room. In some cases, I've heard that people don't even see the doctor! Fortunately, there are some things you can do to keep the doctor in the room a bit longer to answer your questions. Most importantly, step up to your role as your loved one's advocate and physical therapist.

First things first, when you ask a question, get out a notebook and a pen and write it down. If you don't think that you have the correct spelling or information written down, ask! This is so important and common sense, but common sense often goes out the window when there is massive stress involved.

It is critical that you learn the art of listening. The doctors have a limited time to work with the patient and their families, unfortunately. Don't mess it up by talking too much, telling stories about yourself or your dog and monopolizing the doctor's time. If you try to keep the doctor in the room, they will think twice before they come back.

Be professional. Act like an advocate or therapist. The process of hospital to home happens really fast and has gotten worse with the new Medicare guidelines. It's also always helpful to have a second set of ears. If possible, have someone with you for all meetings.

Care plan meetings, where the staff meets with the family to discuss the care and future of the residents in their rehab center, can make you anxious and feel intimidated, but don't let them upset you. The care plan meeting is to make sure that everyone is on the same page. Each meeting usually includes a member of the medical staff, the social worker, the dietitian, a member of the rehab team, and a member of the activities department. It can feel overwhelming but you must remember that they are there to help you work through the process. Don't be afraid to ask questions, point out problems that you see are arising, and review medications and diet-related needs.

There will also be financial meetings, discharge planning meetings, and sometimes rehab staff meetings. It is your right to observe the rehab department as they work with your loved one. This will give you some insight into the deficits and how you might support the rehab process. If you don't understand something, ask!

Meetings are an important part of navigating the healing process. But should you include your stroke survivor in them? You are their advocate, so it's best to protect them by letting them recover in peace. It is not mandatory that your loved one be present in the meetings, but it is important that they are part of their own care and they know what is happening to them and around them. It's natural for anyone to want to protect their loved one, but it's not always good practice to keep information from them. At the same time, use good judgment to not upset the stroke patient by telling them about issues that are beyond their control.

Be aware that if your loved one does attend a care plan meeting and there is a member of the rehab staff present, it is most likely that the meeting time will count toward the allotted rehab minutes for that day. In other words, if your stroke survivor has sixty planned physical therapy minutes for that day and the care plan meeting takes thirty minutes, your loved one will only get thirty minutes of physical therapy exercise for the day.

This is such an important topic that I've dedicated an entire chapter to it, so turn to chapter 7 for more guidance on effective communication.

## THERAPY FOR YOUR LOVED ONE: MEDICAL JOURNAL

The final piece of guidance is something we already introduced, but it bears repeating. It's so important to keep a good medical journal. It helps with the retrieval of information, and is a great reminder of what has been communicated between the family and medical staff. For more information on how to keep a medical journal or to download medical journal forms, see the Appendix or go to www.kathinaumann.com.

---

3 www.chopra.com

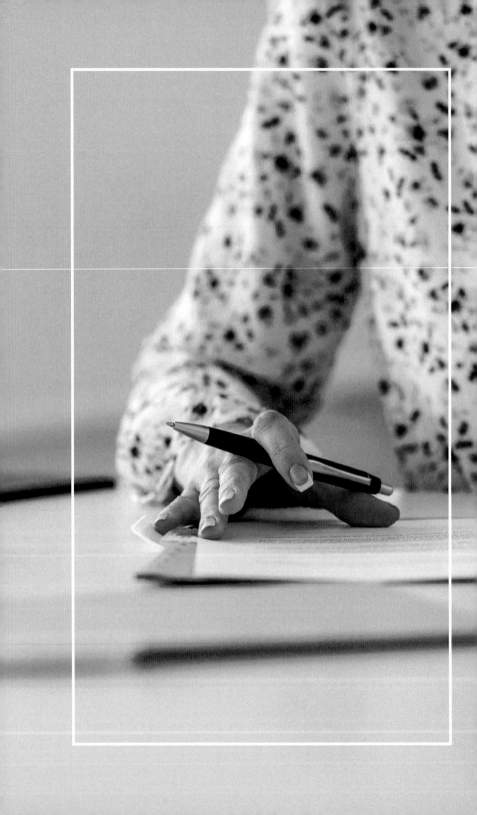

# CHAPTER 3

# LEGAL PAPERWORK
# (COMMON ADVANCE DIRECTIVES)

---

*Although it is still early in your loved one's recovery process, you'll need to be prepared to deal with the legal side of this unfolding situation. It's scary to think that we have the power to decide the fate of someone else, but there are times we must consider the quality of life of someone in need. When Dad had his stroke, I believe it was about forty-eight hours later when the first social worker approached us about signing a do-not-resuscitate (DNR) order. It was all so overwhelming and shocking. Everything was happening so fast, it was hard to process it all. A DNR is a legal form that means if your loved one needs cardiac pulmonary resuscitation (CPR), the medical staff will be obligated not to do it. A DNR is one of the many legal forms called common advance directives.I hope that you find this list of common advance directives helpful and gives you a chance to absorb the next weeks and months to come. It's hard for many of us to talk about dying. Some people are worried that if they talk about death with someone who has a serious illness it will take away that person's hope. This is a hard topic but a very necessary conversation that will make the situation a bit easier.*

**Living Will:** A document that sets out how someone wants to be cared for in an emergency or if they are incapacitated. A Living Will is a document that explains whether or not a person wants to be kept on life support after becoming terminally ill. This is the first document that should be created to ensure that a person's medical wishes are honored. Try to be as specific as possible on this document, but realize that you can't account for every situation that may occur: that is where the POA comes in. The major difference between a will and a Living Will is the timing. A Living Will goes into effect while the person is alive; a will does not go into effect until after a person dies. It is also important to document treatments that you don't want as well as treatments that you do want.

**A living will contains:**
- **Durable power of attorney (POA)**
- **Do-not-resuscitate (DNR) order**
- **Physician's (or medical) orders for life-sustaining treatment (POLST or MOLST)**
- **Organ donation directive**
- **Advance directive for psychiatric care**

To be valid, a living will must be in writing. Some states require that living wills be renewed after a certain number of years.

**Power of Attorney (POA):** A POA, also known as a healthcare POA, is a legal document that identifies who can make decisions for an individual if they are not able to make decisions for themselves. If a person has not selected a healthcare POA, state law dictates who can make healthcare decisions on their behalf if they are incapacitated.

A POA applies any time an individual is incapable of making healthcare decisions for themselves, not just near the end of their life. A healthcare agent may be called upon to make decisions while a person is temporarily incapacitated. If the person you are supporting regains the ability to make decisions for themselves, the proxy's power is no longer in effect. The person who is assigned your durable POA can never contradict the terms of your living will. The POA is there to fill in the gaps for situations that have not been outlined in your living will.

Do-not-resuscitate (DNR): A written instruction from a physician or other authorized healthcare provider stating that a patient should not be given cardiopulmonary resuscitation. It is a legal order usually written/initiated in the hospital to withhold cardiopulmonary resuscitation (CPR) or advanced cardiac life support in respect of the wishes of a patient in the case their heart stops or they stop breathing. A DNR does not affect any treatment other than that which would require intubation[4] or CPR. Things are more complicated if the person has a DNR and they stop breathing or their heart stops while at home, in school, or in the community. Unless the emergency personnel who arrive on the scene are able to find and quickly determine that a DNR is in place and valid, they will perform CPR despite that person's wishes.

Physician Orders for Life-Sustaining Treatment (POLST): Sometimes known as Medical Orders for Life-Sustaining Treatment (MOLST), this is only intended for people with limited life expectancy. The POLST/MOLST spells out specific treatments a patient should receive in an emergency or medical crisis. It is a highly visible, portable document that is kept with the individual at all times, a fully actionable document followed by all emergency personnel that come into contact with the individual. It can be used for the care of a minor. More information on this type of advance care planning can be found on the National POLST Paradigm Task Force Website at www.polst.org.

Organ Donation Directive (ODD): Just about anyone at any adult age (over eighteen) can be an organ donor. To donate your organs after death, you can register at www.organdonor.gov or when you renew your driver's license. Being an organ donor does *not* have any impact on the quality of care you receive while in the hospital.

Advanced Directive for Psychiatric Care (PAD): The Psychiatric Advance Directive is a relatively new legal document that is used to document a competent person's specific instructions regarding future mental health treatments in the event that a chronic mental illness impairs their mental competency. This document must be drafted when a person is well enough to consider preferences during a crisis. In some cases they may authorize an agent to make decisions on their behalf regarding their psychiatric care. Go to www.nrc-pad.org for more information.

---

[4] The process of entering a tube through the mouth into the airway so that the patient can be connected to a ventilator that will force air into the lungs.

---

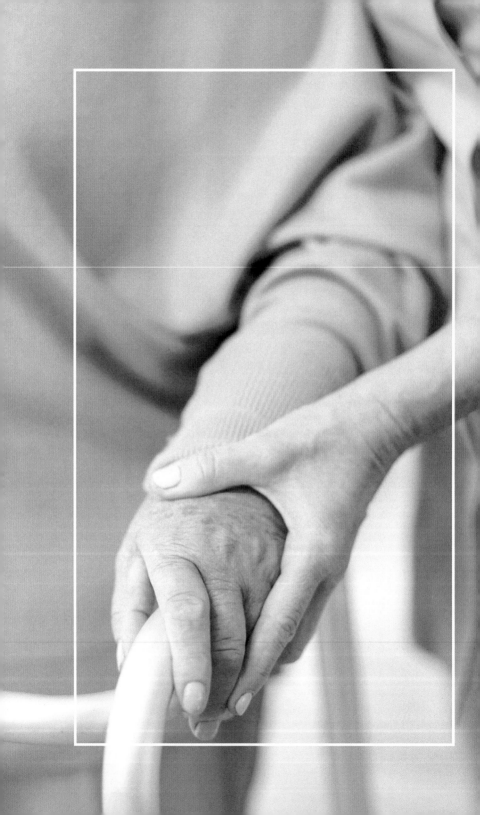

# CHAPTER 4

# REHAB

*The next phase of your loved one's recovery will involve time in a rehabilitation center. There are two kinds of rehab center: short-term (acute care) and long-term (skilled therapy or skilled nursing) rehabilitation centers. I won't lie to you: there's likely a long and difficult road ahead. Later in this chapter I'll share my advice on how to select a rehab center, but first I want to talk a little bit more about some of the challenges we experienced, and what I wish I'd known when my dad started rehab.*

My training as a physical therapist assistant, coupled with my ability to grasp my surroundings, allowed me to understand that my father's inability to focus was going to be a problem. He was there physically, but mentally I could tell he was someplace else. His eyes would be wandering in another direction and he'd be deep in thought while the therapist was giving him tasks to complete. Not one thing is certain when a person suffers a stroke—all strokes are different—but time is a constant, and it was not on our side. Each time Dad "failed" at a task represented less time he was "rehab-able." Patients must show progress for therapy to continue. Dad had just suffered a massive stroke, we were all in shock, his visual field was cut in half, his left, dominant, side was limp and then we were told that most people don't survive this kind of stroke and to expect the worst. Feeling overwhelmed every single day was the norm. Our entire family was living in a state of chronic stress.

Maybe you think by now I am beating a dead horse over this, but taking some time for yourself is crucial. When your loved one arrives at the rehab center, stay close for a few days to hammer down their routine. Once the routine is established, figure out the best time for you to carve out some "me" time.

Most of us mothers feel torn between providing for our children's needs and leaving the home to work. To say that we live a life of constant upheaval in this regard could not be more true when we need to work to survive. Now, I was torn between being there for my four- and five-year-olds, being a wife, selling a house and supporting my parents as they traveled unknown territory. We were starting over with a new set of rules. If I could have been torn in two or cloned myself, that would have worked out just fine. The rehab hospital was located almost two hours from our home. Life was not easy—and I can truly imagine your life is not either, or you wouldn't be reading this book right now. Stay laser-focused, and don't assume anything. This might be a good time in your life to read the book *The Four Agreements: A Practical Guide to Personal Freedom*, by Don Miguel Ruiz with Janet Mills. It will help.

## WHAT TO LOOK FOR IN A REHAB CENTER

Okay. Enough of my story. Let's dive into what you really need to know about searching for short-term and long-term rehabilitation centers.

## ACUTE CARE SHORT-TERM REHABILITATION

Short-term or acute care rehab is just that: short-term. The average stay for acute

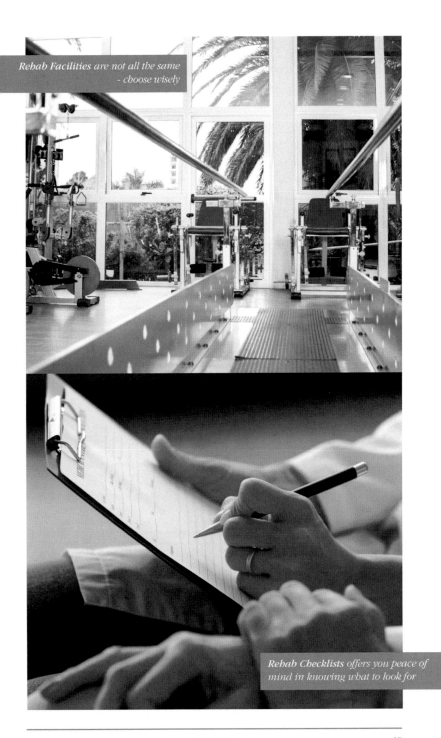

*Rehab Facilities are not all the same - choose wisely*

*Rehab Checklists offers you peace of mind in knowing what to look for*

rehabilitation, according to the American Speech-Language-Hearing Association, is twenty days. You can find more information about levels of care at www.asha.org. Short-term rehabilitation centers are typically run efficiently, and the time you spend there will be fast-paced. You will receive clarity around your loved one's health and given advice and opinions—and this is when reality will most likely strike.

Most of the stroke recovery seems to happen at this stage, but by no means think that recovery ends here. It is actually only the beginning. Keep a positive attitude, no matter what you are told. I have a lot of respect for doctors, but I also know they are not psychic, do not have crystal balls, and certainly are not higher beings—and they are going to tell you the worst-case scenario most of the time.

## CHOOSING A LONG-TERM (SKILLED NURSING) REHAB CENTER

Choosing the right rehab facility could be the most important decision you make. No pressure here, then!

First, muster up some deep strength. Do not get hung up worrying about what others might think of you when you go into a nursing home or rehab setting—ever! The bad news is that this is hard, but the good news is that your decision-making skills and control of the process will increase the likelihood that your stroke survivor continues to improve. It's very important to ask questions, even if it makes the nursing home staff a little uncomfortable. But do it in a kind and caring way. Remember that the people working in these facilities are typically caring people who are overworked and underpaid. Your situation is not their fault, so don't treat them like it is.

Focus your time and energy on picking the right long-term rehab center. It's where you will be spending a lot of your time, and your loved one will be living there all the time. Strike up a conversation at the grocery store, ask the lady at the post office: word of mouth is the best source of information when it comes to choosing a rehab for your loved one. Choose wisely, so that you will have peace of mind when you leave the rehab at night. You need to know that your loved one is being taken care of.

If the rehab knows you're paying attention, they will also pay attention. What I mean is that when the staff of a nursing home understands that you have a higher standard in what you expect from them, they typically rise up and deliver. Be kind and humble, and it doesn't hurt to bribe them a bit too. Occasionally we would bring in a bowl of plums with packs of gum sprinkled inside and a little note that read, "Thanks for taking such good care of our dad." The employees appreciated the notion, and we appreciated the extra care he got.

## REHAB CHECKLIST

In the Appendix you'll find printable pages that contain a checklist of questions and things to look for when searching for a long-term care rehabilitation center. Here they are for your reference as well.

1. What to ask the tour guide
2. What to ask the nursing staff
3. What to ask the rehab staff
4. Things to observe quietly

There are also PDF files for each section available at www.kathinaumann.com. Print them out for each facility you plan to visit and place them on a clipboard to take with you.

These forms were designed to help you get laser-focused and clear about what you want, what you expect, and how you can actually help the staff help your loved one. These are real questions that deserve real answers, so make sure not to move onto the next question until you are completely satisfied with the answer, and don't forget to write things down. When you take notes, the nursing home staff realizes that you are serious. You are serious, but in a non-threatening way. When we're upset and overwhelmed, it's hard to absorb new information (and this is true for anyone!), so be sure to write down all the answers.

There's one more important rule when you're touring a rehab center, which is *don't make an appointment*. Show up unexpected, and ask for a tour. As you enter the facility, talk to other visitors and ask them how their experience is going. You will get valuable information this way. Talking to other people will give you great insight. Do this before you even enter the building, if possible.

Your tour guide is usually the admissions director or someone who works in that department. Remember that their job is to acquire new clients into their system. Nursing homes are also profit centers. Healthcare in the US is a business. They will

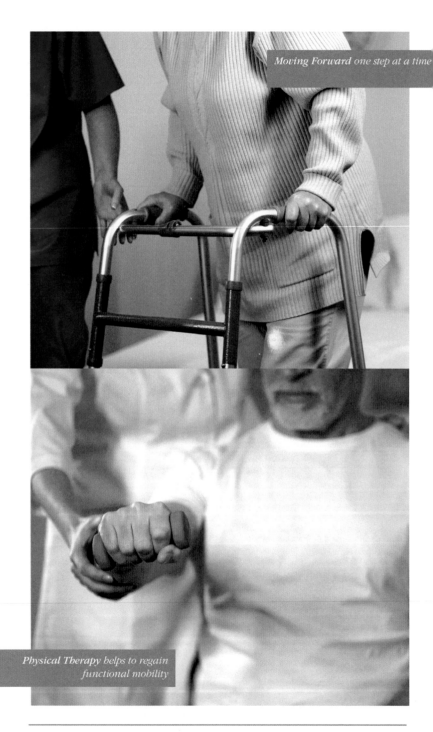

*Moving Forward one step at a time*

*Physical Therapy helps to regain functional mobility*

try to impress you—it's their job. Just remember that you're there to find the best placement for your loved one. The level of care and rehabilitation they receive at this level is critical to their recovery. Your loved one's recovery pays the price if you place them at the wrong facility.

The questions below are aimed to help the person who has no idea what to look for in a rehabilitation facility. They will help you make a well-informed decision about any rehab setting.

## TOUR GUIDE QUESTIONS

1. Do you have a bed available?
2. What are the visiting hours?
3. Is there a doctor or nurse practitioner on staff, and how often do they come to the rehab?
4. What is the name of the rehab company?
5. Are they a contract in your building, or does the nursing home own the rehab company? Many times the rehab department is a contracted company inside a skilled nursing facility or nursing home. Most of the time it doesn't matter whether the rehab company is a contract company, but there are some unwritten perks to having the rehab company employed by the nursing home. Respect comes to mind: when the rehab is part of the entire healthcare team, there is typically a camaraderie between nursing, social work, and the rehab. When we learn to respect one another and work together, the outcome is exponential.
6. Do you have a physical therapist that is certified in neuro developmental techniques (NDT)? For more information on this type of certification, go to www. ndta.org. This is a very special and rare certification, but one well worth asking about. The therapists I know who hold this certification get amazing results. Ask the therapists when you take a tour if any of them have experience working with stroke patients. If they say no, it will not be in the best interest of your loved one, even if the nursing home is around the corner from your home.
7. How many state deficiencies did you have at the last state survey? What were they? Nursing homes that participate in Medicaid and Medicare are required by federal law to undergo an annual survey and certification process by their state health department. Nursing homes must be in compliance with Medicaid and Medicare requirements and state law. Nursing home regulations require that each survey be readily available. If the survey finds a nursing home is deficient because it doesn't

meet a requirement of the federal nursing home regulations, the "deficiency" is recorded on a state survey form.

**8. Do all rehab patients have electric beds?** This may sound archaic, but even in today's life of luxury, electric beds are not always a given. When a person has difficulty moving around, repositioning for comfort, electric beds are a must.

**9. How many private rooms are there, and what is the policy for obtaining one?**

**10. What activities can your loved one participate in, and what do they offer?** Is there someone who supports my family member in getting to these activities if there is not a family member present? This will also give you a sense of commitment from the facility.

**11. Is there a respiratory therapist on staff?** Occasionally, a stroke survivor might need respiratory therapy. The role of a respiratory therapist is to perform respiratory care modalities that include oxygen therapy, breathing treatment, humidity-aerosol therapy, pulmonary draining procedures, mechanical ventilation, and cardiopulmonary resuscitation.

**12. Do you have a full-time speech therapist?**

**13. How does your center measure quality of care?**

**14. Can family be a part of therapy?** Will we be taught exercises and transfers? Education for the patient/family/caregiver is key in building your confidence for managing the basic needs of your loved one. Don't let the transfer from wheelchair to toilet at home be the first time you've ever transferred your loved one. Get a good feel for helping with transfers while still in the rehab center.

**15. Is there a community computer available for the patients to use?**

**16. Can you accommodate a special dietary request?** If your loved one requires a special diet, make doubly sure that you communicate their dietary needs well. For example, let's say your loved one has been getting their nourishment from a tube that has either been placed in their stomach or down through the nose in the hospital, and the day has come to be transferred to acute care rehabilitation. At the new rehab center, your loved one gets their first meal, and it's solid food on a tray. This is when you must ask if the physician's order has been changed, or if this is a huge mistake. These things really do happen. They are not intentional and may cost you the health of your loved one. Hypothetically, let's say your loved one ate the sandwich, which they coughed down—literally. It's very possible that the food did not go down the esophagus to the stomach but down the trachea to the lungs, causing pneumonia. Question everything. It's okay, and it's your right.

---

## NURSING STAFF QUESTIONS

These questions will most likely be answered honestly by the staff if the tour guide is not present—just saying.

**1. Do you like working here?**
**2. How many patients do you care for in one eight-hour shift?**
**3. Is there a registered nurse (RN) on duty 24 hours a day?**
**4. How often are the patients showered, and are the sheets changed at that time?**

## REHABILITATION STAFF QUESTIONS

**1. Observe: Are the staff happy? Laughing?**

**2. How many mat tables are there in the gym?** A center that focuses on neuro development will usually have mat tables lined around the gym/rehab room. Mat table exercises can be especially beneficial for stroke rehabilitation.

**3. How often will my loved one have rehab?** Five, six, or seven days a week?

**4. Do you offer therapy in the morning and afternoon?** Will my loved one have a written schedule? If the answer is "We do what they can tolerate," pay close attention that your stroke survivor is getting the therapy that they need and deserve. An organized rehab schedule is important for routine and recovery. At one rehab my father was in, we would transport him to the rehab for speech therapy, and sometimes we would wait up to two hours for the therapist to emerge from her office. Sometimes she never did.

**5. How many therapists are employed here?** How productive are they required to be? Some rehabs expect their therapists to spend 90 percent of their day being productive in patient care. From a therapist standpoint, this is nearly impossible to achieve while still providing the therapy that the stroke survivor needs and is entitled to.

**6. How many patients do your therapists care for each day?**

**7. How many skilled nursing beds are there in total?**

**8. How many other (different payer source such as Medicare Part B or private insurance) patients do they see?**

**9. Ask to meet the rehab manager. Are they friendly, organized, experienced, and respected?**

## THINGS TO OBSERVE QUIETLY

1. **Is there an odor?**
2. **Are the rooms/hallways clear?**
3. **What does the food look like?** Does it look appetizing? Look at the menu to ensure they serve fresh fruits and vegetables.
4. **How is the food served?** On a tray served in patients' rooms or is it served home-style and everyone eats in the dining room? Socializing is one of the pillars of brain health and recovery. Make every effort to have your loved one eat in a social setting so they don't feel isolated and alone. Maybe they will meet someone who is going through the same life experience and become friends.
5. **Is there access to an outside patio?**
6. **Are the people friendly?**
7. **Are there family members actively participating in patient/therapist treatment sessions?**
8. **Is the staff interacting with the residents and calling them by name?**
9. **Is the equipment in good working order?** Look at the equipment (wheelchairs, walkers, etc.) and take note of their condition. If your loved one is confined to a wheelchair, it's important that the chair fits their needs, and has a cushion, leg rests (unless they can use their legs to propel), and working brakes.

After you've narrowed down the search for a rehab center, ask another person to "pop in" and critique the rehabs for you. It's a good idea to have another person's perspective.

Go to www.kathinaumann.com to find PDF files that can easily be printed and placed on a clipboard when touring a rehab facility.

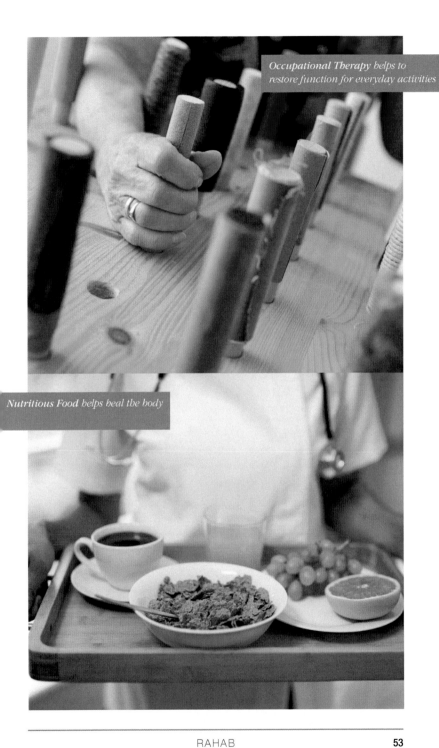

*Occupational Therapy helps to restore function for everyday activities*

*Nutritious Food helps heal the body*

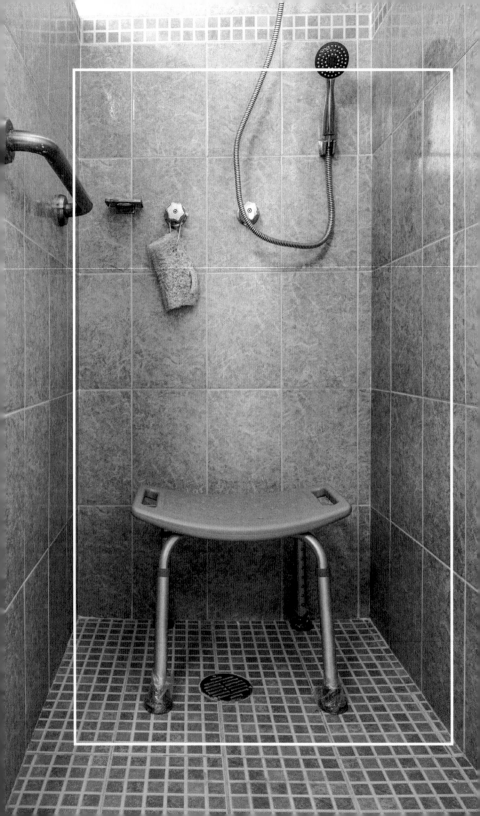

# CHAPTER 5

# THE HOME

*Most people have a desire to remain in their homes rather than move to a nursing home or other facility as they grow older, and I'm one of them. I have worked in nursing home/ rehabilitation centers for almost thirty years, so my opinion comes from the heart. Bring and keep your loved one at home if possible. My parents' home did not have a downstairs bathroom or bedroom when Dad moved home from rehab. We took the dining room table out and replaced it with a hospital bed. Mom gave him bed baths, and once a week we would bring him to our house to take a shower. We had to build a ramp to get him in the back door and squeeze one person, a wheelchair, and a caregiver into our powder- room-sized downstairs bathroom that had no grab bars. Fortunately, Mom and Dad had two wonderful neighbors, John and Earl, who worked endless hours and built them a handicap bathroom on the first floor. They divided the garage and built him a beautiful bathroom with a walk-in shower. I hope John and Earl know how much we appreciate what they did for us. This chapter will tell you what options are available to help you get your loved one home and keep them there.*

## COSTS

It costs on average $83,000 annually to live in a semi-private room in a nursing home. The average cost of $19 per hour for private help at four hours per day equates to $27,0000 annually to stay in your home with help. Twenty-seven thousand dollars to stay in the comforts of your own home vs. eighty-three thousand to live in a nursing home is a no-brainer! I vote to stay at home, and obviously you do, too, or you wouldn't be reading this chapter.

Let's get started! If finances don't allow for private help, make an appointment with social services as soon as possible. They will be able to guide you in creative ways to help support your decision to bring your loved one home. Keep in mind that if Medicaid is your only option to pay for nursing home care, they may ask for their money back at the end of life. My grandfather unfortunately was placed in a nursing home for the final days of his life. Medicaid required payment for the amount they paid out for his care.

### Getting Started with Home Modifications

The American Disability Act is a great place to find information if you are adapting a commercial building or need to cater to the general public. For our purposes, we are adapting someone's personal space so that they can function in that space.

There are five types of design:
1. **Barrier-free.** This type of design was created to help war veterans return to work. It resulted in national standards for barrier-free buildings.

2. **Accessible.** This could be described as the minimal level of design required to meet the needs of people with disabilities. The American Disabilities Act standard is an example of accessible design.

3. **Adaptive.** Adaptive design is used when the construction of a dwelling can be adapted easily down the road, such as placing extra joists for grab bar placement that may be needed later on.

4. **Visitability.** When an environment is created so that a wheelchair-confined person has barrier-free entry and can access the entire first floor and bathroom without difficulty.

**5. Universal.** The new trend in design, popular in large part because our 65-and-older population is the largest it has ever been in the US. Universal Design is used to reduce the physical barriers for people with or without disabilities.

The **universal design model** is the ideal model to use. Maybe you're thinking, "Why is she telling me this?" I am telling you this in case you may be in the position to hire someone to design a handicap space for you and your loved one. If you are not in the position to hire a designer, knowing what design model to use helps when narrowing down your internet search.

Why is universal design ideal? It has six qualities:
- Provides equality for all
- Accommodates right- and left-handed people
- Is simple and intuitive and accommodates a wide range of literacy and language skills
- Is easy to perceive by using different modes of communication: visual, verbal, and tactile cues
- Has fail safe features (for instance, on the computer, a box pops up and asks, "Are you sure you want to delete this file?")
- It requires low physical effort and maintains a natural body position

Now let's talk about the specific modifications you can make, and the options and requirements for each one:

- **Adapting stairs**
- **Threshold ramps**
- **Doorway modifications**
- **Lighting**
- **Toilets**
- **Bidet seats**
- **Power rising toilet seats**
- **Grab bars & railings**
- **Shower & bath solutions**
- **Smartphone Measurement Apps**

## ADAPTING STAIRS

### Considerations
Have two railings that are 1¼" in diameter. Extend the railings 12" past the first and last steps. Treads should be smooth and level. Place a light switch at the top and the bottom. Use a bright light bulb or under-tread lighting. If ambulating stairs are not an option, a stair lift may be the answer. There are standard and custom options available.

### Websites
Bruno.com
Savaria.com
Wheelchairnet.org for tips and an overview of stair lifts
Costhelper.com an excellent site that offers help on thousands of topics

### Costs
Stair lifts start at a do-it-yourself level of $1,000 and can range upwards of $20,000 for custom engineering.

### Who Pays?
Medicare does not cover the cost of stair lifts. An insurance company may cover all or part of the costs. The National Association of Area Agencies on Aging can help you find resources for adults

## THRESHOLD RAMPS

### Considerations
Threshold ramps make traveling over an uneven threshold safer and easier. When determining the length of the ramp remember: every inch of threshold height should equate to 1 foot of ramp length.

### Websites
Pviramps.com
Discountramps.com
Adaptiveaccess.com
Accessibleconstruction.com

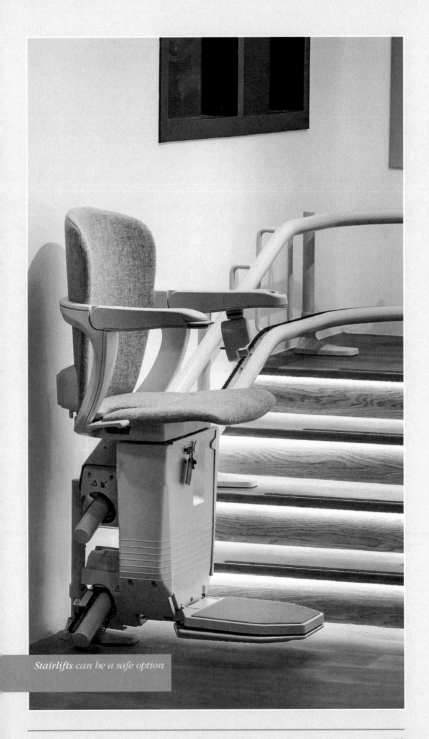

*Stairlifts can be a safe option*

## Costs

Ramps range from $100 starting price for a portable ramp on and up for a custom wood ramp and deck.

## Who Pays?

Medicaid waiver and VA programs cover the cost of threshold ramps. Many long-term care insurance policies also cover the costs of ramps. Habitat for Humanity and other Humanitarian programs will usually build ramps.

## DOORWAY MODIFICATIONS

### Considerations

When measuring for door clearance, always consider that if there is a door in the doorframe you must measure from the opened door to the frame. In other words, measure the clear space, not the door frame.

Options to increase clear door space:
- Off-set hinges
- Remove the door stop
- Enlarge the doorway (if option available)
- Use a lever door handle for easy and simple use
- Use a power door opener (costs approximately $2,000 installed)

### Websites

Adaptiveaccess.com
Monroehinge.com
Accessibleconstruction.com

### Costs

Costs vary from free to approximately $300 dollars for an experienced carpenter to widen a doorway. Hinge prices vary.

### Who Pays?

It is illegal for a landlord to stop a tenant from adapting a rented home for clear access. However, the renter must be able to return the dwelling to its original state. All adaptations are the responsibility of the tenant, unless other arrangements have been made. Use common courtesy, and inform your landlord of any changes that you feel need to be made to their home. A homeowner is responsible for costs accrued to make adaptations to the interior of their home.

## LIGHTING

### Considerations
Having enough light can make all the difference where safety is a concern. If you are wondering if you have enough light, consider purchasing a lux meter, which measures the intensity of the light.

Lux levels for common tasks:
• Kitchen general – 300
• Kitchen Counter – 500
• Bedroom – 300
• Bathroom – 300

Lighting options to consider that will make life easier for your stroke survivor are:
• Slide switch
• Touch lamp converter
• Converter to remote control
• Motion detector lights
• Paddle switch in front of lamp
• Light strip (can use lock adhesive to attach)
• Smart plug to use with a smart device such as an Echo Dot or Alexa

### Websites
Lightinguniverse.com
Amazon.com

### Costs
Touch lamp converter $10
Slide switch $6–$8
Remote control outlet converter $16
Motion detector lights varieties from $20 to $50
Light strip 15 foot $15

**Who Pays?**
Lighting options are not covered by Medicare or private insurance. All lighting is paid for by the consumer.

## TOILETS

**Considerations**
When searching for a toilet, look for "comfort height" or "right height" options, as they ease the on/off transfers. Comfort height are 16" to 17" in height. Elongated toilets are more comfortable for men. Round toilets allow more room in tight spaces. Wall-hung toilets (the tank is mounted inside the wall) allow for the toilet height to be adjusted to the stroke survivor and allow for more space around the toilet.

**Websites**
Amazon.com
Americanstandard-us.com
Plumbingpro.com

**Costs**
Around $300

**Who Pays?**
Medicare and Private Insurance do not pay for toilets.

## BIDET SEATS

Bidet seats are a great option for someone who has difficulty cleaning themselves up.

Bidet is a French word for pony. It comes from the notion that one rides a bidet much like a pony! Despite appearing like a toilet, it would be more accurate to compare it to a wash basin or bathtub. As you can imagine, this could be an invaluable benefit for someone who cannot physically get into a bathtub.

**Considerations**
Most bidet seats require an outlet, but there are a few non-electric options. For cleaning purposes, the wall around the bidet should have larger tiles with less grout.

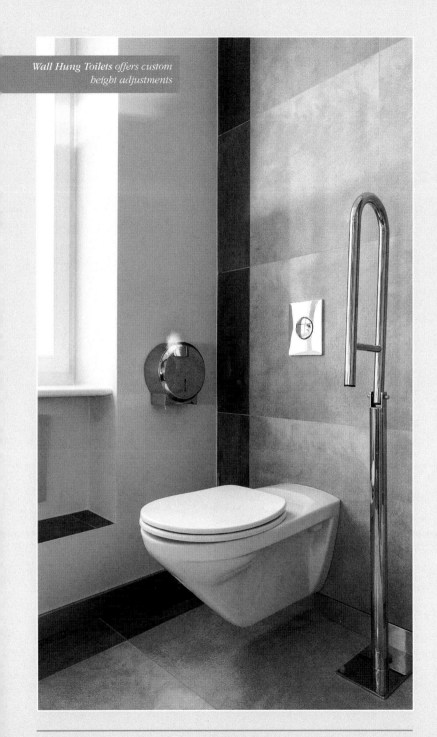

*Wall Hung Toilets offers custom height adjustments*

**Websites**
Cocobidet.com
Kohler.com
Americanstandard.com

**Costs**
Non-electric $75
Electric $250 to $400

**Who Pays?**
Medicare does not pay for bidet seats

## POWER RISING TOILET SEATS

Perfect for the stroke survivor who is having trouble getting up off the toilet.

**Considerations**
Powered rising toilet seats use an AC plug, however battery options are available

**Websites**
Tushpush.com
Liftseat4home.com

**Costs**
$1,200

**Who Pays?**
Medicare and private insurance do not pay for powered toilet seats.

## GRAB BARS & RAILINGS

It's much easier to accommodate the stroke survivor rather than try to ask them to change an old habit, such as reaching for the soap dish or pulling on the towel bar for support. Fortunately for the fashionista, there have been great advancements in grab bars. Grab bars that look and feel like towel bars are available.

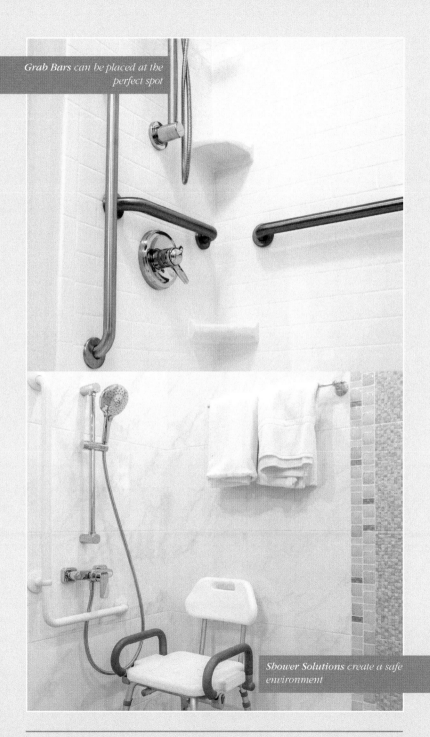

*Grab Bars can be placed at the perfect spot*

*Shower Solutions create a safe environment*

**Types of grab bars**

Wall-mounted

Floor-mounted

Vertical

Adjustable

Angles

**Websites for decorative grab bars**

Csi.moen.com (consulted with Physical and Occupational Therapists)

Amazon.com

Wingits.com

Homedepot.com

Lowes.com

Akw-medicare.com (fold up grab bar)

Healthcraftproducts.com (floor to ceiling bar/pole & angle railing)

Assessibleconstruction.com

**Costs:**

Decorative grab bars range between $30 and $50

**Who Pays?**

Medicare does not consider grab bars a durable medical equipment need, therefore does not cover grab bars; however, private insurance may, so it's worth asking.

## SHOWER & BATH SOLUTIONS

Taking a shower or bath is a risky business when someone has suffered from a stroke. They may have balance and vision deficits, and that coupled with water could be a recipe for disaster.

### Considerations

There are many options to consider where bathing is concerned. If you need help determining which is the best and safest option to get your stroke survivor into the bathtub or shower, consult an occupational therapist. An occupational therapist is trained in energy conservation and best practices for activities of daily living. They can give you pointers for safe ways to transfer a loved one into the shower or tub.

### Transfer solutions for tub options
Bath boards
Transfer benches and seats
Wall-mounted transfer benches
Built-in seats
Portable Bath lifts

### Websites for walk-in shower options
Moen.com (hand held shower and clip)
Homedepot.com (walk-in tube Safeway safety step)
Accessibleconstruction.com (collapsible threshold dam)

### Websites for bathtub transfers
Pattersonmedical.com
Eaglehealth.com
Arcat.com
Ucanhealth.com

### Costs
Costs vary considerably due to the nature of the shower install project
Transfer benches $50 to $100
Wall-mounted transfer benches $50 to $500
Portable bath lifts $1,300

### Who Pays?
Medicare does not pay for transfer benches or any other shower/tub necessities. Fortunately, transfer benches can be found at yard sales. Often your local American Legion gives away medical equipment, so check there first and you may be pleasantly surprised.

## SMARTPHONE MEASUREMENT APPS

Bubble Level
My Measures and Dimensions Pro – take a photo and add dimensions
Photo Measures
Dimensions Pro

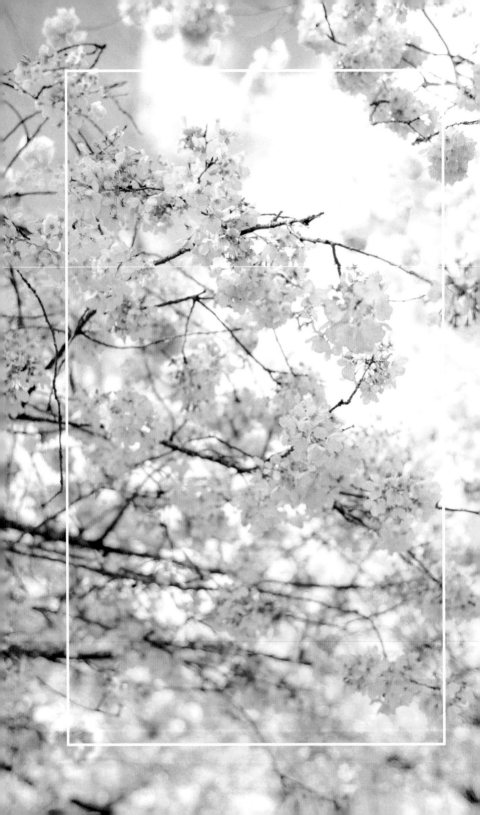

CHAPTER 6

# ALTERNATIVE THERAPIES

---

*Alternative, according to Merriam-Webster, means "different from the usual or conventional." To say that we used alternative means to heal our father would be completely accurate. I grew up planting a garden every spring with my paternal grandfather and harvesting eggs, fruit, and vegetables for my maternal grandmother. I quickly learned that the sun gave me energy, that digging in the dirt grounded me, and that watching the sky gave me information about the weather. But it wasn't until 2005 when my own healing journey began. The Institute for Integrative Nutrition taught me that there are other, sometimes more effective methods to achieving health. Graduating as a Holistic Health Coach gave me the confidence to research complementary and alternative medicine (CAM) to help others and evolve my own health, and I was able to "try" different foods and methods on my father.*

Can you imagine what it was like for me, the daughter of a stroke survivor, to have to learn to catheterize my own father? On one hand, I knew it had to be done for his health, and on the other hand, it was embarrassing and humiliating for us both. Fortunately, as he was being discharged from the rehab center I learned about the alternating hot and cold under the scrotum technique to promote the flow of urination and it worked! My prayers were answered, and so it began... we opened our minds and our hearts to the possibilities that nature and the universe has the ability to heal.

Be aware, though, that some practitioners are reluctant to suggest CAM to their patients. This may be because conventional doctors practicing today did not receive training in CAM therapies so they may not feel comfortable making recommendations in this area of medicine. Some patients are reluctant to mention it to their conventional medicine doctors for fear of being ridiculed. Keep an open mind and an open dialogue with the doctors, and you might be surprised at how many doctors support CAM therapies.

The National Center for Complementary and Alternative medicine now called The National Center for Complementary and Integrative Health (NCCIH), found online at nccih.nih.gov. This US government organization conducts and supports research and provides information about health practices and products. Although there are many evidenced-based research studies on CAM therapies, there are still many unanswered questions about their validity. Do your homework and gather as much information as possible before starting any new medical routine, either traditional or nontraditional.

Often, Dad would suffer from the side effects of the medication he was prescribed, outweighing the benefit of the drug itself. He responded best to natural remedies, so we tried as often as possible to support his healing journey using complementary and alternative methods. The following list of CAM therapies will give you an idea what is available today, but as you do your own search, you may find other alternative methods not listed here.

## ACUPUNCTURE

Acupuncture is a 3,000-year-old healing technique of Traditional Chinese Medicine. Typically, at your first treatment the acupuncturist will take a comprehensive health history, look at your tongue, feel your pulse, and do other physical exams. Using the information from these unique assessment tools, the acupuncturist will recommend a treatment plan. When beginning acupuncture, you lay comfortably on a treatment table while precise acupoints are stimulated with very thin, solid needles. Don't worry—most people don't feel a thing. This part of the treatment may last from five to thirty minutes. Traditional Chinese Medicine practitioners believe that there is a flow known as "qi" or "chi" that is located in certain "meridians" in the body. Chi is what is thought to be the difference between sickness and health, and when the chi is not balanced, illness, pain, poor sleep, and fatigue can all occur. Acupuncture points tend to be where nerves enter the muscle, the midpoint of a muscle, or at the point where muscle joins the bone.

Dad did acupuncture for about four months. I cannot honestly say that it helped with the "pins and needles" he experienced, but it certainly helped with his ability to stay focused and aware. It was similar to someone waking up in a calmer state.

## AROMATHERAPY/ESSENTIAL OILS

Aromatherapy has been used as an alternative for over-the-counter and script drugs for some people. Aromatherapy, also known as essential oil therapy, can be used for medical conditions, ailments, illnesses, and diseases, including stroke. Essential oils are natural oils that are extremely potent and typically obtained by distillation. Oils are good for increasing focus and decreasing anxiety and can help your patient ease into accepting the space they are in and the reality of now. For more information, visit www.naha.org.

## BOTOX FOR PAIN

Botox is a poison that can paralyze nerves, and botox injections have been tried for the management of pain as well as headaches. The theory behind using Botox is that it interrupts the signals that go from the nerves to the muscles and increases the range of motion (ROM). I found a doctor that used Botox for pain and took Dad to investigate it. At the first treatment we were told all the possible side effects and the dangers of Botox. I remember turning to Dad and saying, "Are you sure you want to do this?" He replied, "Yes, I want to try it." I guess I never truly understood how much pain Dad was actually in, because the list of side effects scared the hell out of me, but for him he saw a chance to get out of pain. Don't get me wrong: he complained, but I think he must have had a high threshold for pain. The Botox treatments did not cure the pain in his foot; however, he did notice a decrease in the "pins and needles" that he experienced in his left hand.

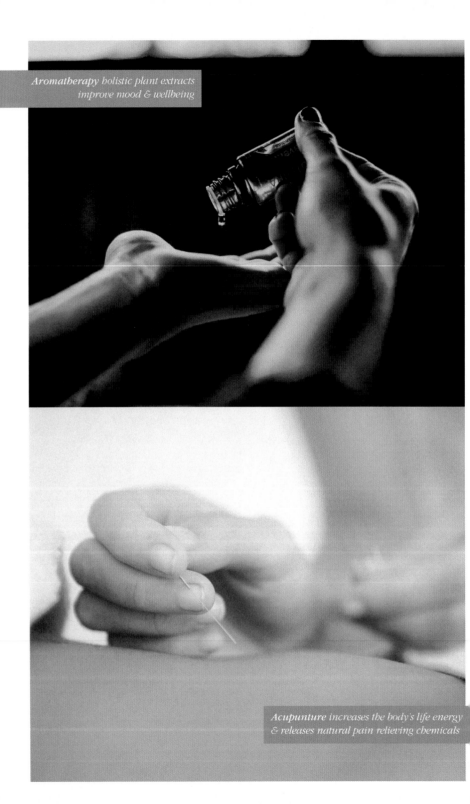

*Aromatherapy* holistic plant extracts improve mood & wellbeing

*Acupunture* increases the body's life energy & releases natural pain relieving chemicals

## CBD OIL FOR PAIN

Cannabidiol (CBD) is a compound found in cannabis and hemp plants. Hemp has been used for centuries to make textiles such a clothing and rope. It creates an indestructible product. To keep things simple, think of it this way: A house is made of lots of building materials that we'll call compounds for this analogy. And the same thing goes for plants—there are many compounds that go together to make a plant. One of the compounds in cannabis and hemp is THC, and another compound is CBD. THC is what we know makes us high if we smoke cannabis (marijuana). CBD oil is not the compound that makes you high, according to sources. Hemp and cannabis CBD oil does contain THC, but hemp contains less than 0.03 percent of THC, to make it legal. Therefore, CBD oil does contain THC, but not enough to make you high. It's important to understand this in case you are a nurse or other healthcare worker who gets drug tested and you are rubbing CBD oil on your stroke survivor without using gloves.

CBD oil has been proven to help with pain as it decreases inflammation. I am a physical therapist assistant who uses CBD oil with the clients I massage, and I can tell you that it works. In most cases the clients become pain-free, and some notice a decrease in their pain level. I think that anything that decreases pain is worth a try. For more information go to www.nationalhempassociation.org.

## FELDENKRAIS METHOD

The Feldenkrais Method is a gentle exercise program based on principles of physics and biomechanics and an understanding of human development. Feldenkrais stimulates the brain to create new neural pathways to promote communication between the brain and tissues in the body. It has been proven to increase range of motion and improve flexibility and coordination through gentle movements and directed attention. This is a great option for those who want or need to increase their range of motion, work through pain, and create healthier movement patterns. For more information go to www.feldenkrais.com.

## GOAT YOGA

The Goat Yoga Movement started in 2016 in Oregon. Small goats play and climb on you while you perform yoga moves. It's a great way to connect with nature and a form of interspecies interaction—or is it that traditional yoga needed to be spiced up? Possibly the weight of a goat on your back reminds you of the burdens we carry, but on the other hand, the lightness of the goat is a great reminder that things are not as heavy as we might think. If you do decide to do this type of yoga (which, by the way, I secretly think is awesome), don't tell anyone! For more information go to www.goatyoga.net.

## HYPERBARIC OXYGEN

It was once thought that brain cell damage was irreversible, but this is not always so. During a stroke, only a small area of the brain actually dies. The surrounding tissue is injured but not necrotic (dead). It receives some oxygen from peripheral arteries but not enough to keep it fully alive and healthy. Hyperbaric oxygen revitalizes this injured tissue and sometimes restores it to full function.

Hyperbaric oxygen therapy can produce a successful turnabout in most stroke patients,[5] and we saw a significant change in Dad. I am not convinced that our father noticed it, but his family sure did. This type of therapy delivers pure oxygen to the patient, and when used within the first twenty-four hours after a stroke, there are cases where after-effects never manifest. Even when the treatment is used years later, a dramatic improvement can be seen. Lingering symptoms can disappear; in fact, people who have tried every other form of treatment to no avail often find success with hyperbaric oxygen therapy.

I have to admit, we tried this form of alternative therapy with Dad to try to ease his left foot pain and heal his brain enough that he would be able to ambulate functionally. Unfortunately, that never happened for him, but what did happen was very subtle improvements. He started to look left occasionally, he was more alert to his surroundings, he seemed happier, and his childlike behavior started to subside. There were times before his oxygen treatments that I felt he was not able to pay attention or stay on task, but after his treatments he was more focused and observant. Purely anecdotal, yes, but the mental clarity was so much that we drove two hours each way for the treatments.

## MENTAL IMAGERY

Mental imagery, also called motor imagery, is the act of "jogging" the brain in the absence of the actual movement, just by imagining it. Studies have shown that imagery of the movement activates the same brain areas that are activated when movements are actually performed.. There is evidence that patients' beliefs that they have control over their recovery predicts the amount of motor recovery achieved. This type

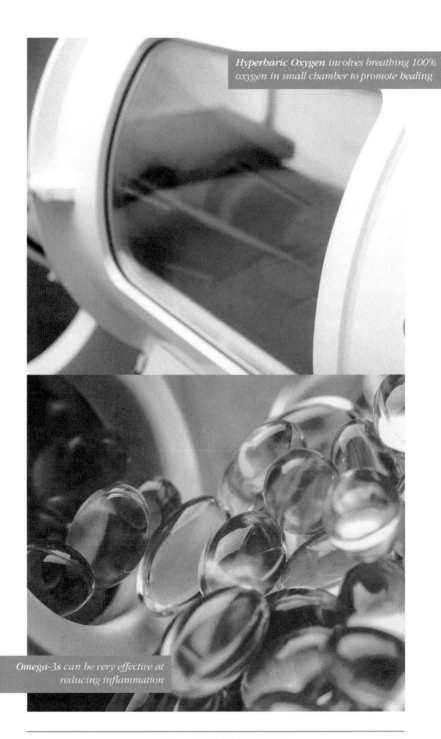

*Hyperbaric Oxygen involves breathing 100% oxygen in small chamber to promote healing*

*Omega-3s can be very effective at reducing inflammation*

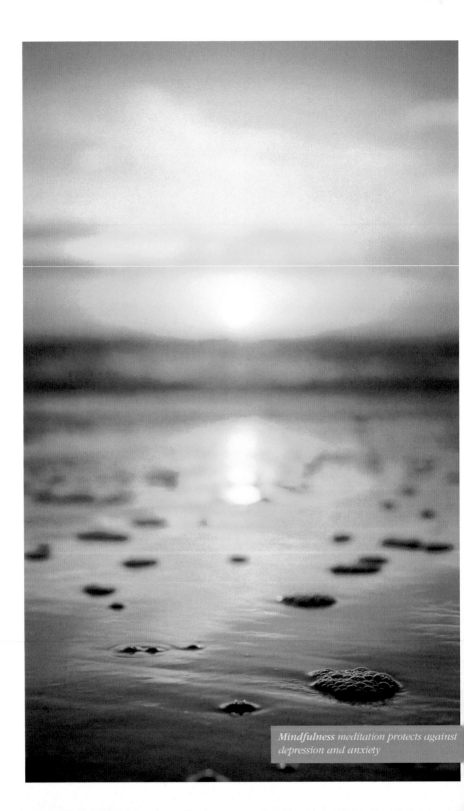

*Mindfulness meditation protects against depression and anxiety*

of mental practice is an attractive rehabilitation option as it would allow patients to practice motor tasks frequently and safely.[6]

## MINDFULNESS

Mindfulness is a form of meditation and a great way to calm the mind. Think of the brain as a puzzle, and during recovery the stroke survivor's mind is trying to put the puzzle back together. A great way to do this is by practicing mindfulness. Have your stroke survivor sit or lie down in a comfortable position. Start the session with an explanation of what you will be doing and why you're doing it. Mindfulness can be performed at any time, but the morning is a great time to practice as it helps get your thoughts together and focused for the day. Think about it: When we're born, the very first thing that we do is take a breath, and when we die the very last thing we do is take a breath, so I'd say that breathing is pretty important. Start by telling your loved one to get comfortable, and close their eyes if they'd like. If they would rather leave their eyes open, have them take a light gaze. Ask them to take a deep breath through the nose and exhale through the mouth. By breathing in the nose and out of the mouth, our bodies and minds gather a sense of peace and a message that everything is going to be okay. If you want to delve farther, I'd suggest Jon Kabat Zinn's books or upload a mindfulness app on your smartphone.

## OMEGA-3S

The omega 3 fats found in a fish oil capsule lower inflammation and can help with a wide range of health conditions. Studies have shown that they can improve your cardiovascular health, lower high blood pressure, lower bad or LDL cholesterol and age-related eye disease, are great for skin, moisturize from the inside out, have anti-aging effects, and reduce fine lines and firm skin. They can help to prevent breast and prostate cancer and maintain healthy tissue. Let's not forget the immense benefits for your brain. These oils have always been known as brain food, and for good reason. They are crucial for maintaining healthy membranes and ensuring nerve signals are sent out with speed and clarity.

## POWER BRAINING

Power BRAINing is a revolutionary, scientifically based program designed to enhance balance, coordination, circulation, processing, focus, memory, physical reaction time, flexibility, and motor control. It is a fitness program that is streamed from the cloud, and an excellent way to spend quality and productive time with your loved one. I love this program! My only wish is that it was available when Dad needed it. You'll need a streaming device such as a TV, computer, or iPad and high-speed internet. I actually offer Power BRAINing group exercise classes in my area, but there is an excellent at-home option. Contact me at kathi@kathinaumann.com if you need more information or would like to get set up with the home version, or visit www.kathinaumann.com. The home version of the Power Braining class is great for the stroke survivor who finds it difficult to enter and exit their home; however, socialization is extremely important to brain health.

## RANGE OF MOTION: YOGA

Range of motion (ROM) is needed to prevent a contracture when the extremity is weak and unable to move in the full range. The muscles in the weak arm or leg will gradually shorten and tighten if the muscle does not get stretched fully several times per day. This is the absolute least a stroke patient should demand of themselves every day.

Yoga helps to increase flexibility, strength and improve posture. The poses help to stretch the muscles, allowing better movement and less stiffness. Yoga can improve balance in stroke survivors who no longer receive rehabilitation care. Fortunately, modern technology makes yoga easier to participate in. Search for yoga apps in your app store or do a simple Google search for yoga videos. There are tons of free videos on the internet these days. Why not take advantage of free stuff?

## REFLEXOLOGY

This is a type of massage that involves applying different amounts of pressure to the feet, hands, and ears. It is based on a theory that these body parts are connected to certain organs and body systems. People who practice reflexology are called reflexologists.

There is one reflexology pressure point that I find to be particularly helpful in calming people who are anxious. The union valley pressure point can be done without the stroke survivor even realizing it. Simply hold their hand in a gentle and calming way and place gently pressure at the union between the first finger and the thumb. With your finger and thumb, gently place pressure for about ten seconds at a time on the "web." Reflexology gives only temporary relief from anxiety, but hey, it works!

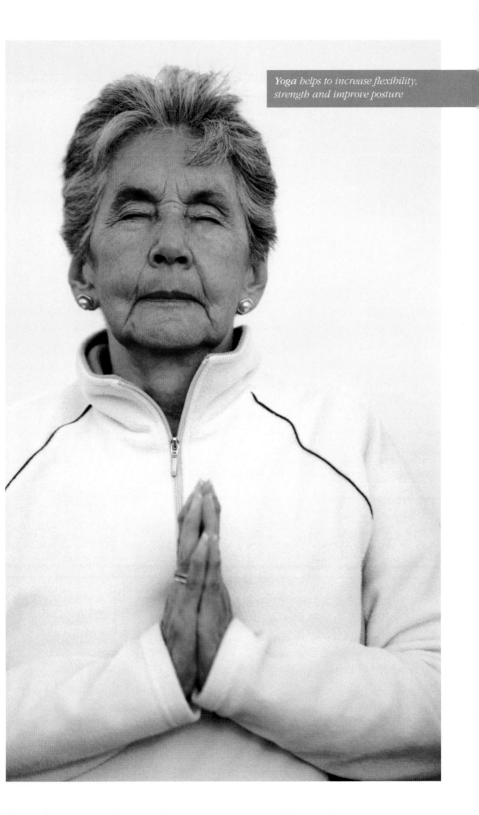

*Yoga* helps to increase flexibility, strength and improve posture

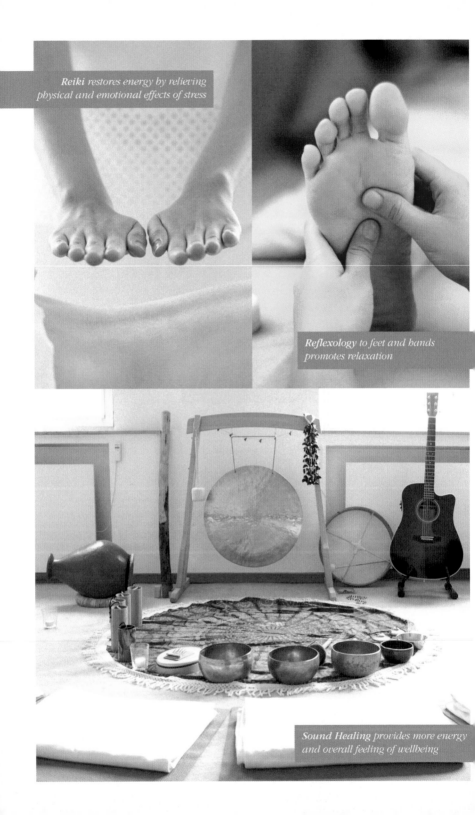

*Reiki* restores energy by relieving physical and emotional effects of stress

*Reflexology* to feet and hands promotes relaxation

*Sound Healing* provides more energy and overall feeling of wellbeing

## REIKI HEALING

Reiki healing uses energy to heal the mind, body, and spirit. Reiki is a relaxing, holistic treatment where natural healing vibrations are transmitted through the hands of the Reiki healer. The Reiki healer acts as a conduit to the body of the recipient. The purpose is to release emotional blockages, relieve stress and pain, induce relaxation, accelerate the natural healing process, and balance the body's energies. Everything on the planet has a vibration. Even the planet itself has a vibration. When we are sick or sad, we vibrate at a lower frequency than we do when we are feeling positive and happy. Reiki healing may raise the body's vibrational frequency and promote healing. The International Center for Reiki Training estimates that there are four million people throughout the world who have taken at least one level of Reiki Training. Today, Reiki education is offered in more than 800 US hospitals. For more information, see www.centerforreikiresearch.org/Downloads/HospitalListTable.pdf and www.centerforreikiresearch.com.

## RELOX: BRAIN NUTRITION

Couple hyperbaric oxygen with a new discovery and you might just be on to something good. Relox is a nutritional IV therapeutic technique developed by Bruce Rind, MD. It consists of an intravenous infusion of a vitamin–mineral solution with the simultaneous application of oxygen by mask. The technique was designed to refresh, oxygenate, and "wake up" brain cells that are still alive but not fully functional. For more information go to www.drrind.com. Dr. Rind's clinic is located in Maryland.

## SENIOR FITNESS MEMBERSHIPS

Typically, the order goes something like this: hospital, acute rehabilitation, long-term rehabilitation, home care, outpatient therapy, fitness memberships. Many gyms offer a maintenance-type exercise membership for seniors with disabilities. Also, your outpatient physical therapy office may also have a program established for people who no longer need the benefit of a skilled service. Some states also offer the Silver Sneakers program that is covered by Medicare. It's worth looking into.

## SOUND HEALING

Sound healing is a noninvasive, natural form of vibrational energy medicine. It has the power to heal our wounds and ignite our spirit. For thousands of years, sound has been successfully used as a powerful healing tool. There is an abundant amount of research supporting the healing properties of sound. The mind-body connection has taken a sledge-hammer to a once carved-in-stone dogma with its new discoveries. Backed by a stack of countless studies, we now know that our cells' ability to dominate disease and protect against foreign invaders is under direct command and control of the mind. For more information go to soundhealersassociation.org.

## STROKE CAMP

Stroke Camp is a camp for stroke survivors and their caregivers. Typically, they participate in arts and crafts, camp songs, good food and company, bonfires, games, fishing, boating, and hiking. In the US, there are more than seven million stroke survivors. Stroke Camp is a place for stroke survivors to go to feel normal again—to feel that they can do the things they once did before they suffered from a stroke. Dad never attended a stroke camp, but I know that if he had he would have loved every minute of it—he was an adult male with the heart of a kid. For more information go to www.strokecamp.org.

## VISION THERAPY

Vision therapy is a type of physical therapy for the eyes and brain. It usually is a highly effective treatment for many common visual problems such as lazy eye, crossed eyes, double vision, convergence insufficiency, and some reading and learning disabilities. Many patients who have been given little hope have benefited from vision therapy.

There are eye doctors who practice eye therapy, and there are internet programs available. Dad attended eye therapy in Bethesda, MD, where he performed activities that strengthened his mind and his eyes. He actually liked his eye therapy sessions. He suffered from hemianopsia, where half of his visual field was cut, and sadly, that did not return. We were told that his eyesight would not return, but we had to try. This therapy was well worth the time and money involved.

Vision therapy uses a metronome, which helps with neurotiming, hand-eye coordination, and balance. The metronome gave him auditory feedback to know whether he was in sync, allowing him to make corrections to improve timing and rhythm. For more information, visit www.neuroeyecoach.com or do a Google search for eye therapy.

Watching Dad try to find an 8x10 piece of white paper sitting on the table in front of him was one of the hardest moments in my life. Sometimes these little moments really hit home and make us realize that nothing is ever going to be the same. How the hell did this happen and why is it happening to me? To us? To our families? It just isn't fair.

Dad's stroke happened just around the time cellphones started to become a thing. I didn't have a smartphone with a metronome app, so I had to make one. Hitting a wooden spoon on the table to give a rhythmic tune seemed like a good enough way, and so it all began.

I typed random letters in bold size 72 font, printed them, then hung them on the wall directly in front of him. It took about three sessions of me physically putting his head in a neutral midline position before he actually understood that there were letters on the wall. The letters looked something like this:

| P | H | D |
|---|---|---|
| T | A | B |
| Q | E | R |
| N | G | X |
| O | K | J |

Each time I hit the table with the spoon, Dad was supposed to say a letter. At first we worked in a downward motion, then as he got better at it we started reading the letters from left to right. This was extremely difficult for him, and many times he gave up. Occasionally, there were even tears in his eyes. Fortunately for him, he had support and a daughter who was determined to teach him to read. All my determination, along with his will to be able to read to his grandchildren, came together and made a spark so large that he eventually went on to read out loud at a weekly Bible study. I was so proud of him.

Overall, the vision therapy helped with his attention, processing speed, motor coordination, reading fluency and comprehension, motor coordination, and expressive language skills. I felt that the vision therapy moved him forward in his healing process more than any other therapies in this chapter.

---

5 www.ncbi.nlm.nih.gov/pmc/articles/PMC4420971/

6 Find more information in this article: https://www.ncbi.nlm.nih.gov/pmc/articles/PMC2797860/

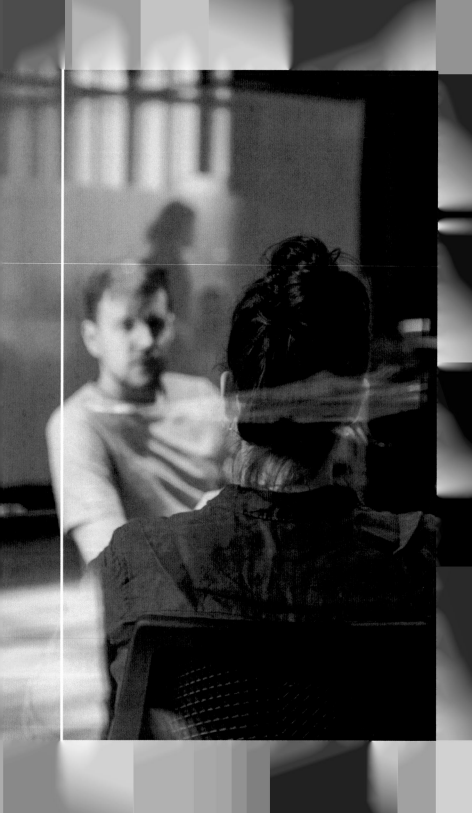

# CHAPTER 7

# EFFECTIVE COMMUNICATION

*Learning how to communicate effectively is a life-long journey, and is especially important to learn when you want to gather as much information as possible about your stroke survivor in the fifteen minutes the doctor has to spend with you. Actually, if you get fifteen minutes, consider yourself lucky. According to a 2016 study by CRICO Strategies, healthcare miscommunication cost the U.S. $1.7 billion and 2,000 lives. Good communication is not hard to do, and it's critical that you learn how to communicate with the staff. If you know you're not a good communicator, find someone in your family who is while you learn this skill. I'm serious here. Good communication skills are a must in this fast-paced recovery process. You want and need the healthcare team on your side. In this chapter you'll be taking a crash course in communication. Pay attention and read this more than once. The goal of clear communication between the caregiver (unfortunately, that's you!) and the doctor is to get the best outcome for your stroke survivor, period. Learn these simple but very effective communication strategies and receive the best care possible for your stroke survivor.*

## INTRODUCTIONS

Always introduce yourself to whomever. Make it laser clear to the medical staff what your relationship is to the patient. For example, start out your introduction like this, "Hi, my name is Kathi, and I'm John's oldest daughter." Let the staff know your role. Are you the decision maker? If not, who should the staff refer to? Repeat this every time someone new comes into the room. This will give the healthcare worker a sense of relationship. When someone rents their house, it's good practice to leave family photos around so that the renters will get the feeling that the owner is a real person with a real family and will be less likely to trash your place. This rings true in this situation as well – informing the healthcare workers who you are and your relationship to the patient only strengthens their will to help you. In the medical journal there's a form for the family tree. Print it.

## SUPPORT BUDDY

Have someone else with you at all care plan meetings or meetings with the financial office. Care plan meetings can be overwhelming, but they're really nothing to worry about. A care plan meeting is just a way to make sure that the staff and family members all have a clear understanding of what the plan is and to bring them together to move forward. Typically these meetings are scheduled for twenty minutes. Ask questions and write the answers in your journal.

And do not include your stroke survivor, especially if you know there is a conflict. Protect your loved one by allowing them to recover in peace. This does not mean hiding important information from them, but it does mean using good judgment and not upsetting the stroke survivor by telling them about issues that are beyond their control. They must be calm and feel positive about their recovery process. At home, in the classroom, a factory, an office, and especially in a rehab setting, a learner must feel good about themselves for the learning process to have a chance to work. A human being cannot learn in the real sense of the word if they are hurting, overtired, depressed, frightened, embarrassed, ashamed, angry, confused, or bored. A learner must be feeling good in order to really learn. Sadly, a stroke survivor often feels all these emotions at once.

## MEDICAL JOURNAL

Be prepared with questions to ask before any meetings, and since you started a medical journal, this is exactly where you will write your questions and the answers.

Review the questions just before entering the meeting. Remember, human beings cannot intelligently take in information that they cannot relate to what they already know. If you are not already in the medical field, then all this is very new and overwhelming. If you are not prepared when you enter the room, you could misunderstand or miscommunicate, which might lead to disaster later on. Write down the questions in your journal and write the answers next to them. If you are having trouble understanding what the doctor is saying, simply say, "I apologize, but I don't fully understand." If you are a visual learner, ask the doctor to write down the information about the diagnosis or treatment (this might not work if their handwriting is not the best). You can even have them write it directly in your medical journal.

Another great way to preserve the information is to upload a recording app to your smartphone. Many phones already have this feature/application build in. This way you can go back and listen to the information as many times as you need to; it can also come in super-handy when another relative or friend wants to know what's going on. Ask the doctor if you can record them before you do it.

## LISTENING AND BEING LISTENED TO

Stop and listen. Force yourself to hear. Even if you are quiet for a moment, your head could be swirling with all the things you want to say. Having all your thoughts clearly written down in an organized format gives you, the caregiver, a sense of peace and organization. You can then talk about the information and relate it to what you know.

Information must be presented in small increments for learning to take place. Too large a package of information is as bad as none at all. This occurs simply because the evaluation process is all jammed up by the frustration of not being able to make references fast enough to keep up with the material.

Do not leave any unanswered questions. You have the doctor In your presence, so take full advantage of it. We live in a world of information overload, and that includes the doctor. It is important to get clear on our ideas and to clearly communicate information that is meaningful. Refrain from telling personal stories unless it is absolutely critical information that will change the recovery outcome.

Are you desperate to be listened to? You bet you are, and talking about what is happening right now in your life is good therapy, but it must be done in the proper context. A medical doctor is typically not a psychotherapist, and nothing will make them run out of the room faster than being made to feel like they are one. If you feel a strong need to talk things out, I suggest you go outside and find an animal to talk to, find a friend who will listen, or even talk to yourself. Or schedule an appointment with a psychotherapist, of course!

## BODY LANGUAGE

Pay attention to your own body language (nonverbal communication). Understanding the body language of others is extremely useful, but you must pay attention to the message your own body language is sending. Conflicting body language and words are a recipe for misunderstanding: when your words and body are sending different messages, people will tend to go with body language. Here are the body language rules to follow:

- Do not cross your arms
- Do not look at the clock
- Do not yawn
- Do not face the door as if you can't wait to leave
- Always look the doctor in the eye
- Always smile and introduce yourself by giving your name and relationship
- Always write down the answers to the questions you have
- Always respond politely when referring to information you do not understand
- Always have someone else with you (other than the stroke survivor)
- Always be considerate—remember, doctors are people too, and kindness will go a long way toward getting you the kind of treatment and communication you deserve
- Always be open and honest

## MIRRORING

Use "mirroring" to get clarity. Mirroring is a form of communication that allows you to get very precise with the information you're receiving. If something is unclear to you, try repeating it back to the doctor. After listening to the doctor, reply by saying, "So, I think you are suggesting that..." or, "So, what I am hearing you say is..." or, "So, you mean I should ..." Always use "I" statements such as the ones suggested. It is offensive to point blame at someone else for your misunderstanding. Never say, "You are being unclear," "You are not making any sense," or, "You are using too many medical terms." Instead, you could say, "Okay. What I am hearing you say is ..." or,

"I am sorry but I don't understand what you just said. It is a little complicated for me since I don't have a medical background. Could you please repeat it?"

Understand that when miscommunication occurs, it can create internal conflict. This conflict can burn our willpower and rob us of energy. And energy is not something you can afford to lose right now. Get very clear about the message you want to convey or the answers you want to receive. You must not have guilt or internal conflict about the answers or how you portray them. If you do not feel good about how you have given or received information, let it go and strive to do better at the next meeting. Communication is difficult, and the ability to communicate clearly is critical in life. A small shift in communication can have a powerful impact.

## THE ART OF LISTENING

Now that you are aware of the art of communication and how to speak clearly and precisely, it's critical that you learn the art of listening. The doctors have a limited time to work with the patient and their families, unfortunately. Don't mess it up by talking too much, telling stories about yourself or your dog and monopolizing the doctor's time. If you try to keep the doctor in the room, they will think twice before they come back. Have you ever found yourself avoiding someone because you are on a time constraint and you know they will just make you later than you already are? This is the same concept: most doctors in a hospital setting are on a strict time constraint.

General features of a good listener:
- Approval—look at the doctor with approval.
- Delight—be delighted to see them.
- Respect—treat the doctor with respect.

Almost all distress carries with it disrespect. When someone we love has a stroke, not only do we feel like we've been knocked down, we feel beat down. We feel oppressed, and at the core of all oppression lies disrespect. You may not agree with everything the doctor says, especially when they tell you that your loved one will not get any better. This is so far from the truth it's not even funny, but it happens. You may also receive this message in a nonverbal format. Just remember that miracles do happen: the more you work with your loved one, the better they become—and you can take that to the bank.

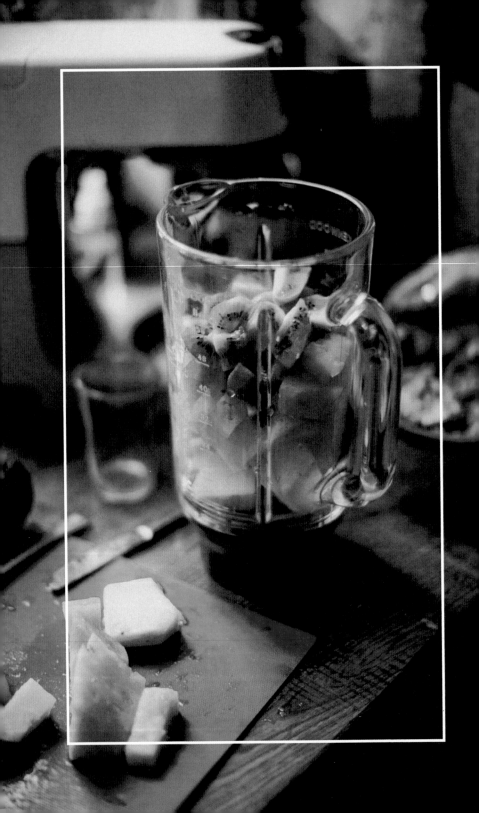

# CHAPTER 8

# RECIPES AND NUTRITION

*I come from a food-as-medicine perspective. I healed myself through good nutrition and mental health habits, and was able to incorporate that same philosophy into the healing of my father through superfood nutrition that took him from a point where he was unable to locate objects lying on the table in front of him to reading out loud at a Bible study once a week. I truly believe it was the good nutrition and alternative medicine that provided him the tools he needed to recover and change his life for the better. Good nutrition and healthy habits will help change the health of your loved one. The trick to surviving this is by staying healthy yourself and perpetuating the healing of others.*

# EAT LIKE YOUR LIFE DEPENDS ON IT! BECAUSE IT DOES...

## BRAIN-HEALTH DIET: SMOOTHIES

Let's get started by unlocking the healing powers of the brain by introducing whole natural foods into your loved one's diet and your own. These recipes were ones I created for my father. These recipes provide much more than necessary calories. They contain ingredients that are essential to improve the health and quality of life of you and your family. Nutrition is our original medicine, and the food we eat can be either the most powerful form of medicine or the slowest form of poison. Those who discover whole foods begin dancing to the beat of a different drum, and as our blood quality begins to change, we start to heal from the inside out.

Make nutritious thickened liquid smoothies instead of those pre-made high fructose corn syrup-laden drinks that can sometimes do more harm than good. Always start with the cleanest, richest-in-color, best-quality foods you can obtain. When grocery shopping, don't just pick up a piece of produce and run off with it. When you enter the store, take a deep breath, and enjoy the moment if you can. Caring for a loved one is overwhelming, and having an excuse to "step out" for a minute is a great way to recharge, even if the grocery store is the best excuse you can find. Take time to heal yourself while purchasing the foods that will heal them, too. Choose the fruits and vegetables that stand out against the rest—the ones with vibrant color, clear of blemishes and bad spots. If you find that you are shopping for a specific item and they all just look blah, don't waste your hard-earned money on it and move on. If it looks blah to you, then it probably tastes that way too. Maybe you have time to stop at another store, or you can adjust your recipe.

Wash all the fruits and vegetables with clean water to wash off the dirt, grime and pesticides. Some people actually wash their produce with soap. There are several vegetable soaps on the market, but I like to use Dawn dish liquid.

I use a Vitamix to make all my smoothies, but any high-speed blender will do. It does not need to be fancy, but it does need to be able to crush ice. Place all the ingredients in the blender, add water, and blend until smooth.

Less water gives you a thicker end result. This is very helpful if your mom or dad has a swallowing problem. Don't be afraid to tweak the recipes to your loved one's liking.

All smoothies can be transported easily using an airtight mason jar and can last up to twenty-four hours in the refrigerator. Food has energy, and your smoothie will have the most energy when it is first made. It will lose its energy over time, just like we do, so it is best to consume it immediately after you create it.

Each recipe contains information on the benefits the ingredients possess. The standard American diet, also known as the SAD diet, does not provide the necessary nutrition to sustain a healthy body. We need to step up our nutrition. We are up against superbugs like MRSA, environmental toxins like cancer-causing Roundup and viruses like Covid-19. Even the smallest amount of high nutrition consumed by your stroke survivor is better than none at all.

## RECIPES TO BUILD STRENGTH, ENERGY & STAMINA

You can't mess up a smoothie, and I dare you to try! (I have messed them up, actually, but only because I don't like super-thick or sour smoothies.) All recipes are intended for a large-size blender such as a Vitamix.

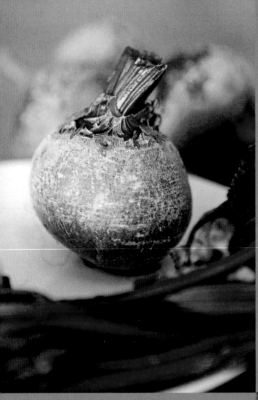

## OXYGEN BOOSTER

*Helps with carrying oxygen in the blood. Great for people with anemia. Beets have a natural blood pressure-lowering quality.*

**2 small beetroot**
**3 beet leaves**
**1 carrot**
**1 apple**
**water to the top**

Wash the beetroot and leaves, carrot, and apples. Place all the ingredients in a high-speed blender and cover with water. Blend well until smooth.

## POWER SMOOTHIE

*Provides a protein punch that'll fuel you with long-lasting energy! Protein helps us to feel full, so this is a great smoothie if you get hungry quickly.*

**3 cups almond milk**
**½ cup fresh or frozen berries**
**½ cup fresh or frozen mango**
**2 tablespoons raw almond butter**
**sprinkle of cinnamon**
**4 or 5 kale leaves**
**handful of spinach**

Wash the spinach and leaves. Place all the ingredients in a high-speed blender and cover with water. Blend well until smooth.

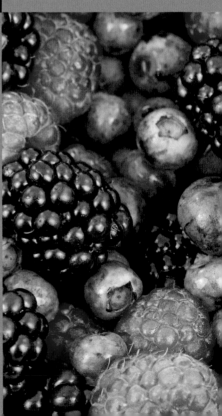

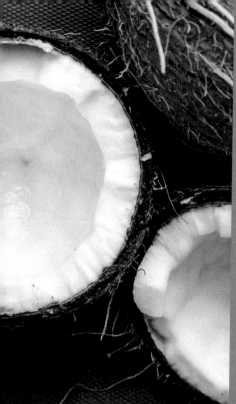

## VANILLA MAJESTIC SMOOTHIE

*Sweetness in a jar—good for the sweet tooth. Sugar is no good for the brain. If you find you need something that curbs the sweet tooth, try cutting back on the sweetener over time.*

3 cups almond milk
1 cup coconut meat
1 whole vanilla bean, scraped or ¾ teaspoon vanilla extract
1 tablespoon coconut butter
2 tablespoons agave or other sweetener of choice (I like stevia powder)

In the high-speed blender, blend all ingredients until smooth.

## DETOX POWERHOUSE

*This contains choline, a nutrient that stimulates the liver. Choline precedes acetylcholine, which is important in memory and muscle control.*

3 green apples, cored & quartered
2 kiwis, quartered (skin on)
3 cucumbers (skin on)
5 kale leaves and stems
6 romaine leaves
1 ½ cups of spinach or dandelion greens

Wash the fruit, veggies and leaves. Place all the ingredients in a high-speed blender and cover with water. Blend well until smooth.

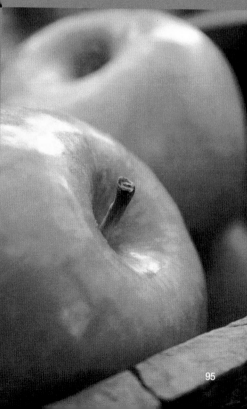

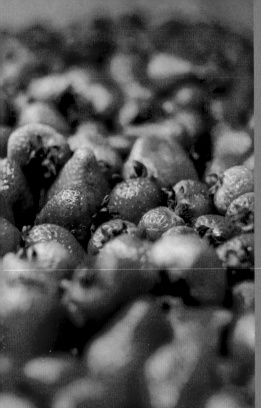

## DELIGHTFUL DESSERT

*Manganese is a mineral that helps heal soft tissue. This sweet drink supports the joints as well as the sweet tooth.*

**2 frozen bananas
2 cups strawberries
½ cup raspberries
2 tbsp stevia
Enough coconut milk to cover the ingredients**

Add ice cubes if desired. Blend and enjoy.

## PEACHY KEEN

*Contains two types of fiber: insoluble helps prevent constipation, and soluble feeds the cells in your gut.*

**2 peaches halved
1 small handful of kale
1 banana
2 tablespoons fresh hazelnuts with skins or Nutella Hazelnut Spread
enough cold coconut milk to cover ingredients**

Blend well.

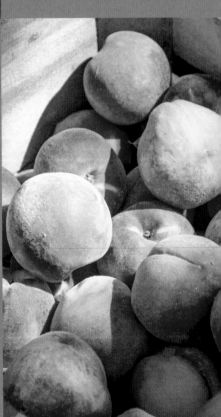

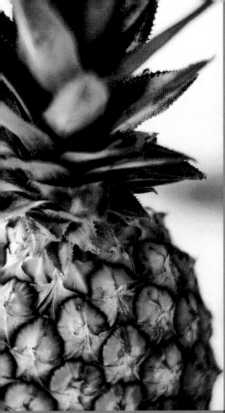

## PAIN RELIEVER

*Pain sometimes comes from inflammation. Foods that reduce inflammation can help in the healing process. All the ingredients have a cooling effect and help to reduce inflammation.*

**1 rib of celery
1 cup of cucumber
½ cup of pineapple
½ of lime wedge (peeled)
enough coconut water to cover the ingredients**

Wash ingredients and blend well.

## BRAIN BOOSTER

*Blueberries have been found to improve communication between cells (yes, the cells talk to each other), enabling you to learn new information faster!*

**1 cup blueberries
1 small banana
½ cup cucumber
1 tablespoon chia seeds
1½ cups fresh water**

Wash the fruit, blend and enjoy.

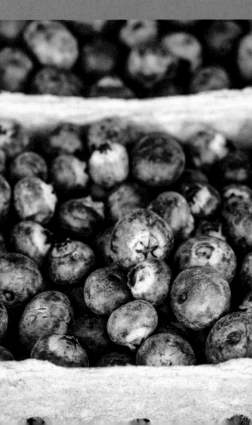

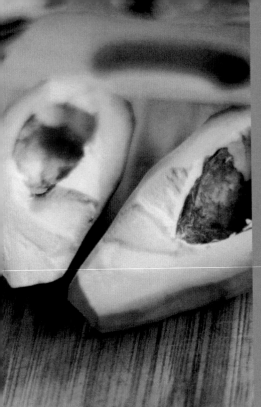

## BACTERIA-BLASTING SMOOTHIE

*This smoothie packs a serious immune system punch that's high in vitamin E and selenium. Vitamin E is needed for healing the skin.*

1 avocado peeled & pitted
2 tbsp brazil nuts
1 tbsp stevia
1 tsp vanilla
fresh clean water to cover the ingredients
ice is optional

Wash the ingredients and blend until smooth.

## NATURALLY THICK PEACH & STRAWBERRY OATMEAL

*Great healthy alternative to Thick-It thickener (a thickening powder used when survivors have trouble swallowing).*

1 peach
6 frozen strawberries
¼ cup rolled oats (cooked)
½ cup plain, fat free Greek yogurt
¼ cup orange juice
1 tablespoon chia seeds
2 ice cubes

Blend well, and don't forget the spoon!

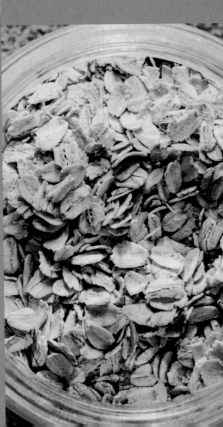

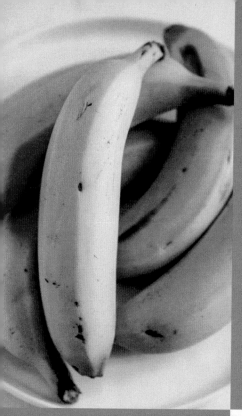

## QUICK & ON THE GO!

*Ovaltine is a high nutrition health drink powder that is caffiene free and suitable for vegetarians. It is high in sugar though so not a smoothie you'd want to consume every day.*

**2 frozen bananas**
**3 tablespoons Ovaltine**
**1 tablespoon organic peanut butter**
**handful of kale**
**¾ cup pure water**

Blend and go!

## IMMUNE-BOOSTING SMOOTHIE

*Avocados are bursting with fiber and help ease constipation.*

**1 avocado**
**1 banana**
**1 cup blueberries**
**1 cucumber**
**a fistful of kale or spinach**
**stevia to taste, and/or a sprinkle of cinnamon or cacao**

Wash the fruit and leaves. Place all the ingredients in a high-speed blender and cover with water. Blend well until smooth.

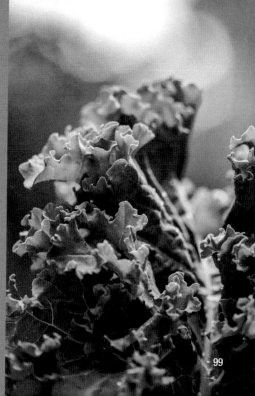

## BRAIN-HEALTH DIET: MEALS

The latest research on brain health focuses on the Mediterranean - DASH intervention for Neurodegenerative Delay (MIND) diet. The MIND diet is a combination of the DASH diet and the Mediterranean diet, in an attempt to create a brain health and health creation type diet.

Dr. John McDougall is a famous nutrition expert and healer, and his website (at www.drmcdougall.com) is a great resource if you are looking for healthy meal plans or would like to attend in-person workshops. Dr. McDougall suffered a massive stroke at the age of eighteen that left him completely paralyzed on the left side of his body for two weeks. He gives credit to eggs, double cheese pizza, and hot dogs for his brain damage—and his good fortune. He claims that If not for his stroke, he would most likely not have become a doctor. He grew up in the suburbs of Detroit, Michigan, in a lower middle class family. His website is chock full of very useful information. Don't forget to read Dr. McDougall's story—it is fascinating.

I understand how overwhelmed you are. Maybe you are thinking that you can't possibly do any of this right now, but try to make just one change in your loved one's diet. Only one is all it takes to get their energy flowing toward health and away from a bad and negative flow of energy. Think of energy as water flowing, and now you've diverted the flow of the water (energy) in a different direction. It's really that easy to change the direction of energy. It's boils down to only one thought: the thought to buy and consume one good-for-you item at the grocery store. Take it home and prepare it. Slow down. You've got this.

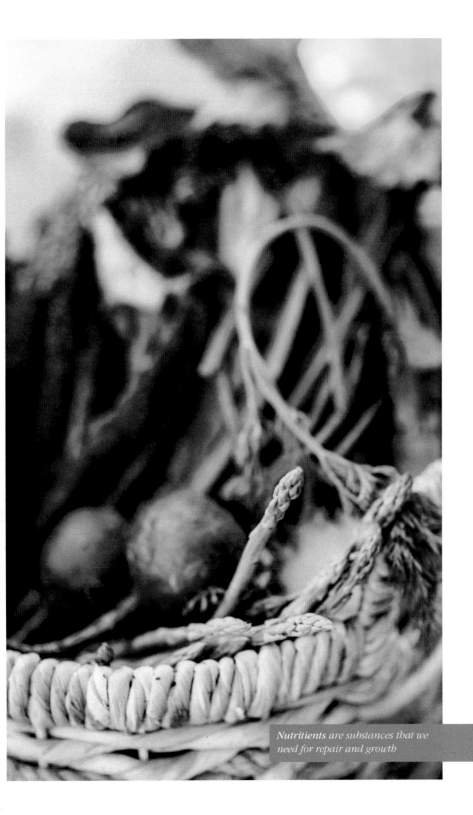

*Nutritients are substances that we
need for repair and growth*

APPENDIX A

# MEDICAL JOURNAL

*A lifeline for caregivers*

PATIENT NAME

........................................................................

## MEDICATION LIST PRIOR TO STROKE

List medications, vitamins and other dietary supplements prior to stroke.

| NAME OF MEDICATION | DOSAGE | TIMES TAKEN PER DAY |
|---|---|---|
| | | |
| | | |
| | | |
| | | |
| | | |
| | | |
| | | |
| | | |
| | | |
| | | |

## MEDICATION LIST AT ACUTE HOSPITAL

List medications taken during acute hospital stay.

Dates: ...........................................................................................................................

| NAME OF MEDICATION | DOSAGE | TIMES TAKEN PER DAY |
|---|---|---|
| | | |
| | | |
| | | |
| | | |
| | | |
| | | |
| | | |
| | | |
| | | |
| | | |
| | | |
| | | |
| | | |
| | | |

## MEDICATION LIST AT REHAB FACILITY

List medications taken during stay at rehabilitation facility/skilled nursing facility

Dates: .................................................................................................................

| NAME OF MEDICATION | DOSAGE | TIMES TAKEN PER DAY |
|---|---|---|
| | | |
| | | |
| | | |
| | | |
| | | |
| | | |
| | | |
| | | |
| | | |
| | | |
| | | |

## CURRENT MEDICATION LIST

List current medications          Date: ................................................................

| NAME OF MEDICATION | DOSAGE | TIMES TAKEN PER DAY |
|---|---|---|
| | | |
| | | |
| | | |
| | | |
| | | |
| | | |
| | | |
| | | |
| | | |
| | | |

## ABOUT THE STROKE

Date of Stroke: ....................................................................................................................

Time of Stroke: ....................................................................................................................

Story of how it happened: ....................................................................................................
....................................................................................................................................
....................................................................................................................................
....................................................................................................................................
....................................................................................................................................
....................................................................................................................................
....................................................................................................................................
....................................................................................................................................
....................................................................................................................................
....................................................................................................................................
....................................................................................................................................
....................................................................................................................................
....................................................................................................................................
....................................................................................................................................
....................................................................................................................................
....................................................................................................................................
....................................................................................................................................
....................................................................................................................................
....................................................................................................................................
....................................................................................................................................
....................................................................................................................................
....................................................................................................................................
....................................................................................................................................
....................................................................................................................................
....................................................................................................................................

## CAREGIVER'S CALENDAR

**Tip:** The caregiver/volunteer schedule listed on a calendar can be very helpful, especially when posted on the patient's bulletin board.

Month: .........................................................................................................................

| SUNDAY | MONDAY | TUESDAY | WEDNESDAY | THURSDAY | FRIDAY | SATURDAY |
|--------|--------|---------|-----------|----------|--------|----------|
|        |        |         |           |          |        |          |
|        |        |         |           |          |        |          |
|        |        |         |           |          |        |          |
|        |        |         |           |          |        |          |
|        |        |         |           |          |        |          |

## HOSPITAL – ACUTE CARE

Name of Hospital: ..................................................... Phone: ................................

Admission Date: .................................... Discharge Date: .........................................

Name of Physician/Title: ............................................. Phone: ...............................

Occupational Therapist: ..................................................................................................

Speech Therapist: ...........................................................................................................

Day Shift Nurse: .................................... Nursing Assistant: .......................................

Evening Shift Nurse: ............................... Nursing Assistant: .....................................

Night Shift Nurse: ................................... Nursing Assistant: ......................................

Housekeeper: ..................................................................................................................

Director of Nursing: .................................................. Phone: ...............................

Assistant Director of Nursing: ....................................... Phone: ..............................

Social Worker/Case Worker: ...........................................................................................

Phone: .................................................. Office Hours: ...........................................

Medical Billing Advisor: ..................................................................................................

Phone: .................................................. Office Hours: ...........................................

## HOME HEALTH CARE

Home Care Agency: ................................................. Phone: ..............................

Initial Date: ........................................ Discharge Date: ..........................................

Name of Nurse/Therapist who opened case: ...............................................................

Phone: ........................................................................................................................

Nurse: ..................................................................... Phone: ..............................

Certified Nursing Assistant: ........................................ Phone: ...........................

Physical Therapist: ...................................................... Phone: ...........................

Physical Therapist Asst (PTA): ...................................... Phone: ...........................

Occupational Therapist: .............................................. Phone: ...........................

Occupational Therapist Asst.(COTA): ........................... Phone: ...........................

Speech Therapist: ...................................................... Phone: ...........................

# IDENTIFICATION CARD

The medical identification card is not only a practical tool for doctor's appointments, it can also be a lifesaving device for your stroke survivor. Fill out the card, print it out, cut & fold in half and place in their wallet.

**Reminder:** As the medications change, update the information on the card and reprint.

## EMERGENCY MEDICAL INFORMATION

**I am a stroke victim. I have Aphasia. I am not drunk.**

My name is: .........................................................................

Date of Birth: ......................................................................

Caregiver's name:: ...............................................................

Caregiver's number: ............................................................

Fold here — — —

## MEDICATIONS

| NAME | DOSE |
|------|------|
|      |      |
|      |      |
|      |      |
|      |      |

**OTHER IDENTIFICATION TOOLS:**
Identification bracelets, emergency flash drives and mobile apps are all practical and possibly lifesaving tools. First responders can have instant access to all your emergency information electronically.

## OUTPATIENT THERAPY

Outpatient Facility: ................................................... Phone: ...............................

Date of initial evaluation: ........................... Date therapy began: ...........................

Physical Therapist: ................................................... Phone: ...............................

Physical Therapist Asst. (PTA): .................................... Phone: ...............................

Occupational Therapist: ............................................. Phone: ...............................

Occupational Therapist Asst.(COTA): ........................... Phone: ...............................

Speech Therapist: ................................................... Phone: ...............................

Date of 30-day re-evaluation: ......................................................................................

Assessment after 30 days: ..........................................................................................

.................................................................................................................................

.................................................................................................................................

Date of 60-day re-evaluation: ......................................................................................

Assessment after 60 days: ..........................................................................................

.................................................................................................................................

.................................................................................................................................

Date of discharge from outpatient therapy: ..................................................................

Date fitness training began: ........................................................................................

## PATIENT INFORMATION

Patient Name: ................................................................................................

Address: ..........................................................................................................

Date of Birth: ................. Religion: ................. Normal Blood Pressure: .................

**MEDICATION**
Medication Allergies: .......................................................................................

..........................................................................................................

Medications the patient has trouble with:

Medication: ............................... Issue: ...............................................................

Medication: ............................... Issue: ...............................................................

Medication: ............................... Issue: ...............................................................

**FOOD**
Food Allergies: ...............................................................................................

..........................................................................................................

Food the patient has trouble with:

Food: ............................... Issue: ...............................................................

Food: ............................... Issue: ...............................................................

Food: ............................... Issue: ...............................................................

**OTHER ALLERGIES & ISSUES**

..........................................................................................................

..........................................................................................................

..........................................................................................................

## REHABILITATION CENTER

Name of Rehab/Skilled Nursing Center: ................................ Phone: ......................

Admission Date: .................................. Discharge Date: ......................................

Name of Physician/Title: ............................................. Phone: ...............................

Physical Therapist: ................................................................................................

Occupational Therapist: .........................................................................................

Speech Therapist: .................................................................................................

Day Shift Nurse: ..................................... Nursing Assistant: ..................................

Evening Shift Nurse: ............................... Nursing Assistant: ..................................

Night Shift Nurse: .................................. Nursing Assistant: ..................................

Housekeeper: ......................................................................................................

Administrator: ........................................................ Phone: ................................

Director of Nursing: ................................................. Phone: ................................

Asst. Director of Nursing: ......................................... Phone: ................................

Social Worker/Case Worker: ...................................................................................

Phone: .................................. Office Hours: .....................................................

Medical Billing Advisor: .........................................................................................

Phone: .................................. Office Hours: .....................................................

## HELPFUL INFO FOR REHAB STAFF

Is patient right-handed or left-handed? ....................................................................

Normal Rise Time: ....................................................................................................

Normal Bed Time: ....................................................................................................

Wears Glasses? .......................................................................................................

Wears Hearing Aids? ...............................................................................................

Hard of hearing? .....................................................................................................

Strongest Ear? ........................................................................................................

Is cognition Impaired? .............................................................................................

Number of steps in home? ......................................................................................

Favorite foods: ........................................................................................................

....................................................................................................................................

Food Dislikes: .........................................................................................................

....................................................................................................................................

Food Considerations: (thickened, diabetic, high blood pressure, requires low sodium,

allergies) .................................................................................................................

....................................................................................................................................

....................................................................................................................................

# PATIENT'S FAMILY TREE

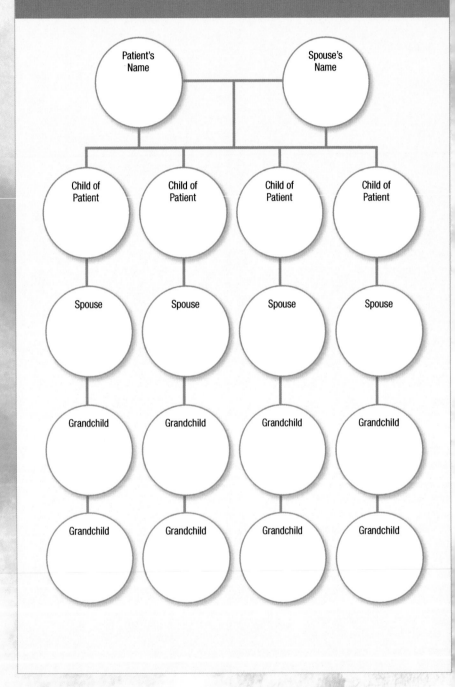

## APPENDIX B: REHABILITATION FACILITY CHECKLIST

Name of Facility: ........................................................ Date: ................................

Name of Admissions Director: ......................................... Phone: ...............................

### QUESTIONS TO ASK THE TOUR GUIDE
Does your facility have a bed available? ...................................................................

What are the visiting hours? ...............................................................................

Is there a doctor on staff & how often do they come? ..............................................

What is the name of your rehabilitation company? ..................................................

Do you have a therapist that is NDT (Neuro Developmental Techniques) certified? ...

..........................................................................................................................

How many state deficiencies did you have in the last state survey? What were they?

..........................................................................................................................

Will your stroke survivor have an electric bed? ......................................................

Ask the tour guide to see an occupied room. Is the bathroom clean and free of odor?

..........................................................................................................................

How many private rooms are there, and what is your policy to obtain one? .............

..........................................................................................................................

What activities can your loved one participate in, and what do they offer? ...............

..........................................................................................................................

### TOUR GUIDE QUESTIONS (cont.)

How does your center measure quality of care? ......................................................

Can the family be part of therapy? .............................................................

Is there a community computer available for patients to use? ....................................

Can the center accommodate a special diet request? .............................................

### NURSING STAFF QUESTIONS

Do you like working here? ........................................................................

How many patients do you care for in one eight-hour shift? ......................................

Is there an RN on duty 24 hours a day? ..........................................................

How often are the sheets changed? ...............................................................

What is the shower schedule? .....................................................................

### REHAB STAFF QUESTIONS

Is the staff happy? .................................................................................

How many mat tables are there? ...................................................................

Is there rehab six or seven days a week? .........................................................

How many therapists are employed there? .........................................................

# APPENDIX B: REHABILITATION FACILITY CHECKLIST

**MAKE OBSERVATIONS**

Is there an odor? .................................................................................................

Are the rooms and hallways clear? ......................................................................

What does the food look like? (Look at the menu to ensure they serve FRESH fruits and

vegetables.) ..........................................................................................................

How is the food served? On a tray in patient's room? Home style in dining room? .......

.............................................................................................................................

Is there access to an outside patio? ......................................................................

Are the people friendly? ........................................................................................

Are the family members actively participating in patient/therapist treatment sessions?

.............................................................................................................................

Is the staff interacting with residents and calling them by name? ..............................

.............................................................................................................................

Look at the equipment (wheelchairs, walkers, etc…) and take note of their condition.

.............................................................................................................................

## ABOUT THE AUTHOR

**Kathi Naumann** is a health educator with a strong affinity for supporting the entire family. She spent the first ten years of her physical therapy career as a stroke therapist and the next eight years she spent as the daughter caregiver of her father. Her ability to share her own experience, knowledge, and compassion is strongest when working with stroke survivors and their families. Kathi understands that physical healing is connected to spiritual and emotional healing, which doesn't stop and start with the loved one who has suffered a stroke: it must also include you, the caregiver. Her dream is to see those who need help and support around stroke using this book and her other tools as a reference.

## ACKNOWLEDGEMENTS

Thank you **Kris Gowl**, PT for teaching me everything you know about stroke recovery. Your knowledge helped to shape my life. Thank you **IIN** & **Joshua Rosenthal** for your vision and to all the special people I met who are now life long friends. To my Husband **Chris** and our amazing kiddos, **Kylee** and **Mitchell** I thank you and love you. You are truly the people that I am most grateful for. Thank you **Jim Thompson**, videographer extraordinaire, for making my life brighter and for your dedication to creating videos that will surely help the readers of this book. **Christi Hetrick**, thank you for creating my logo and so many modules when I thought that this book was actually going to be a website. **Pam Whyte**, thank you for helping to shape my vision with your writing skills and ability to strategize the content of this project. **Scott Allen** of **Self Publishing School**, I thank you for your support and your calming voice. You taught me to keep my eye on the goal and to keep moving forward no matter how long it takes. A huge thank you to **Reedsy** for connecting me to two amazing people: **Ray Sylvester** and **Janis Utton**. Ray, you are not only a superb editor but a kindred spirit that shares the same drive to help people change their lives and see the bigger picture. And then there is Janis. Wow. I love your creative design style. You are the one that made this guide book come to life and I thank you. Finally thank you **Dad**, for teaching me to forgive.